Physical Modalities
A Primer for Chiropractic

Physical Modalities
A Primer for Chiropractic

Paul D. Hooper, DC

Chair, Department of Principles and Practice
Los Angeles College of Chiropractic
Los Angeles, California

With illustrations by Claire D. Johnson, DC, CCSP

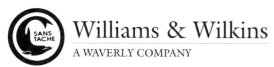

Williams & Wilkins
A WAVERLY COMPANY

BALTIMORE • PHILADELPHIA • LONDON • PARIS • BANGKOK
BUENOS AIRES • HONG KONG • MUNICH • SYDNEY • TOKYO • WROCLAW

Editor: John P. Butler
Managing Editor: Linda S. Napora
Production Coordinator: Raymond E. Reter
Production Services: Marty Tenney, Textbook Writers Associates, Newton Centre,
Massachusetts
Copy Editor: JoAnne Nash
Designer: Marty Tenney
Illustration Planner: Marty Tenney
Cover Designer: Tom Scheuerman
Typesetter: Graphic Sciences Corporation, Cedar Rapids, Iowa
Printer: The Maple-Vail Book Manufacturing Group, York, Pennsylvania
Binder: The Maple-Vail Book Manufacturing Group, York, Pennsylvania

351 West Camden Street
Baltimore, Maryland 21201-2436 USA

Rose Tree Corporate Center
1400 North Providence Road
Building II, Suite 5025
Media, Pennsylvania 19063-2043 USA

Printed in the United States of America

Library of Congress Cataloging-in-Publication Data

Hooper, Paul D.
    Physical modalities : a primer for chiropractic / Paul D.
Hooper ; with illustrations by Claire D. Johnson.
        p.   cm.
    Includes bibliographical references and index.
    ISBN 0-683-04143-6
    1. Chiropractic.   2. Physical therapy.   I. Title.
RZ255.H67 1996   95-42832
615.5'34--dc20   CIP

*The publishers have made every effort to trace the copyright holders for borrowed material. If they
have inadvertently overlooked any, they will be pleased to make the necessary arrangements at the
first opportunity.*

96 97 98 99 00
1   2   3   4   5   6   7   8   9   10

To my wife, Debbie,
who tolerates my disappearing into the computer room
for hours at a time.
and
To Alison and Benjamin,
my biggest fans.

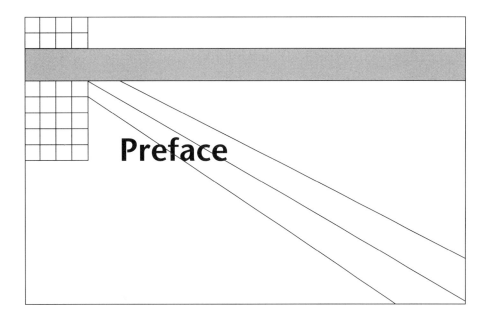

Preface

The use of physical modalities such as electrical stimulation and ultrasound has been commonplace in the chiropractic clinic for many years. While equipment has improved, application techniques have remained fairly constant through the past several decades. The primary purpose of these tools is to enhance the healing process and to reduce the impact of the "vertebral subluxation." Consequently, many of these physical modalities are viewed as ancillary procedures by the chiropractor. So why another text about passive modalities?

Course work in the use of physical modalities is offered in most of the chiropractic colleges and most states require some formal training as a prerequisite to licensure. Currently, there are approximately 15,000 chiropractic students in the world. Annually there are an additional 3,000 to 5,000 students who enroll in chiropractic colleges. In spite of these numbers, there has not been a text written specifically for the chiropractic student.

This text is designed as a teaching aid for chiropractic students taking course work in the use of physical modalities (*i.e.,* Physical Therapy). As such, it is structured to provide a guide that is specifically directed at those modalities and procedures that are common in the practice of chiropractic. The scope of the text includes heat and cold, therapeutic ultrasound, electrical stimulation, microamperage stimulation, traction, splints and braces. The text has several features that make it a unique teaching guide;

- information concentrates on those tools and procedures that are common in chiropractic practice

- chapters and topics are organized in a way to assist the student learning both the physiological basis and the clinical application of each of the modalities
- clearly defined learning objectives assist the student and the instructor
- case presentations and examples are provided

The text addresses the nature of the conditions and problems that are treated with modalities. Throughout, emphasis is placed on the need to develop reasonable treatment objectives based on a clear understanding of the condition in question. Topics covered include the response to injury, the stages of injury, grading soft tissue injuries, and the process of healing and repair. Since the goal of many of the physical modalities is pain control, a review of this important area is provided. Specific topics covered include nociception, pain measurement, and pain control or modulation techniques. Each modality covered includes a discussion of the various indications, contraindications, application techniques, etc. In addition, treatment protocols for specific conditions commonly seen in the chiropractor's office are discussed. Appropriate use of physical modalities in a clinical setting must be based on an understanding of the body's response and proper application techniques.

As we enter the 21st century, the chiropractic profession continues to gain credibility and respect. The case for conservative chiropractic management of many common musculoskeletal conditions is growing. It is hoped that, in some small way, this text may provide the chiropractor of tomorrow with a better understanding of the application of passive modalities in patient care.

Paul D. Hooper, DC

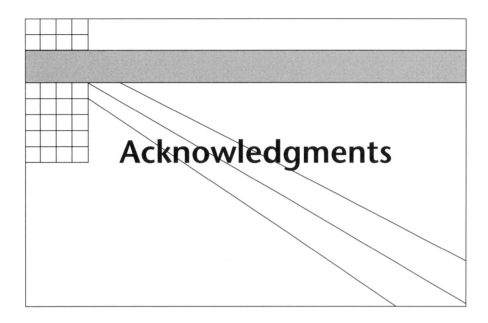

Acknowledgments

There would not be a book without the following people. First, I thank Steve Foreman who started me in the writing business. My thanks, also, to John Butler, who listened to my ideas, encouraged me to continue, and, finally, bugged me to finish; to Linda Napora, who tactfully, but constantly, kept me on target; and to Ray Reter, who directed the production process.

Special thanks to Dr. Claire Johnson for the illustrations and to Drs. Michael J. Stahl and Stephen M. Foreman for their contributions.

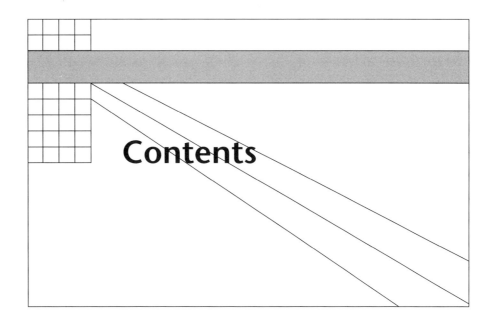

Contents

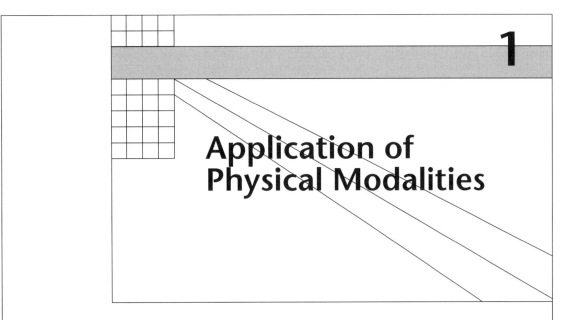

Application of Physical Modalities

Learning Objectives

At the completion of this chapter, you should be able to:

1. Differentiate between active and passive therapy and provide examples of each.
2. Describe the factors that are important in developing a cohesive treatment plan.
3. Describe the inflammatory process:
   - characteristics
   - hemodynamic events
   - cellular events
   - influencing factors
4. Describe the stages of injury: acute, subacute, and chronic.
5. Describe the remodeling process.
6. Describe the deconditioning syndrome.
7. Describe the process of functional restoration, including patient reactivation and work-hardening or activity-specific training.

Manual manipulation of the spine and peripheral joints is not new. Historically, spinal manipulation is one of the oldest treatments for a wide variety of conditions including back pain, neck pain, and some types of headaches. Over the years, spinal manipulation has been used by a number of groups including chiropractors, osteopaths, physical therapists, and some lay practitioners. However, chiropractic is the only profession with such a strong commitment to its use. For nearly 100 years, the chiropractic profession has utilized manipulation as its primary therapeutic tool. In spite of significant opposition, spinal manipulation (*i.e.*, the chiropractic adjustment) has grown in both scope and popularity throughout the world. Although spinal manipulation was once considered unscientific and without any rational foundation, recent evidence supports its legitimate role in the health care system. In fact, currently, the U.S. Agency for Health Care Policy and Research (AHCPR) provides guidelines for the treatment of low back pain. These guidelines, based largely on available research, include the use of spinal manipulation as a recommended treatment modality for patients with acute lower back pain.

Supportive Care: Passive and Active

In addition to relying heavily on the spinal adjustment, chiropractors have long used a variety of other treatment procedures to support or enhance the effect of manipulation. This text looks at the use of some of those additional forms of supportive care for the patient who has or who will have, manipulative therapy. This ancillary or supportive care falls into two primary categories: passive therapy and active therapy.

Passive therapy includes those treatment modalities that do not require any energy expenditure on the part of the patient. Rather, the modalities are applied to the patient while he or she lies quietly on a therapy table. Modalities in this category are very common in the chiropractic clinic and they include manual massage, application of heat and cold, electrical stimulation, therapeutic ultrasound, manual and mechanical traction, and so forth.

Active therapy, unlike passive therapy, demands some active involvement on the part of the patient. Rather than being the passive recipient of therapeutic procedures, the patient must be an active participant in the therapy. Among the active therapeutic modalities are exercise, education, retraining, and work hardening. Current evidence and treatment trends are focusing more attention on active forms of therapy.

As one should realize is the case with any one treatment, manipulation is not a panacea. Rather, it is a means to an end, the end for the patient being the restoration of functional integrity and/or the ability to perform pain-free activities. In many instances, the use of ancillary modalities, both active and passive, is not a luxury but a necessity if the patient is to recover fully from his or her ailment. Ironically, the AHCPR guidelines discourage the use of many of the passive modalities that are discussed in this text. It is, therefore, imperative that clinicians understand the rationale, techniques, and limitations of these treatment modalities. Future use of therapeutic modalities is likely to be based not only on the perceived therapeutic effects, but on outcome measures, cost effectiveness, and weight of scientific evidence.

Goals

Passive Modalities

The use of various physical modalities, such as heat, cold, electrical stimulation, and ultrasound is common in the treatment of back pain and many other musculoskeletal conditions. These modalities are principally effective during the early phases of treatment and are often directed at controlling symptoms such as pain and swelling. Patient participation in the application of these therapeutic procedures is limited primarily to a passive role.

The principal goals for these passive forms of care include:

- relief of pain (*e.g.*, TENS, ultrasound, ice, heat)
- reduction of swelling and edema (*e.g.*, Electrical-stimulation [E-stim], ultrasound, ice, heat)
- reduction of muscle tension (*e.g.*, E-stim, heat, massage)
- improvement of circulation (*e.g.*, E-stim, heat, ultrasound)
- promotion of tissue healing (*e.g.*, E-stim, microcurrent, ultrasound)

In addition to their value during the early phases of care, many of these modalities may prove useful during the more chronic phases of treatment. The goals during the chronic period include:

- relief of pain (*e.g.*, TENS, ultrasound, heat)
- reduction of muscle tension (*e.g.*, E-stim, heat, massage)
- reduction of fibrous tissue and adhesions (*e.g.*, E-stim, ultrasound, massage)
- improvement of range of motion (*e.g.*, E-stim, ultrasound)

Recent evidence indicates that the use of many of these treatment tools may positively affect the healing process and reduce healing times. Both ultrasound and electrical stimulation (especially the microamperage stimulation devices) have been shown to have a similar positive effect on healing times. This may be one of the richest areas both for future research and for developing new treatment applications.

It is important to emphasize that the use of passive modalities is rarely beneficial in and of itself. Rather, they function as a part of a treatment approach. For example, ultrasound is often prescribed for the treatment of tendinitis. Although ultrasound has a number of beneficial effects, it is not particularly helpful if used alone. However, the decrease in pain that often accompanies the use of ultrasound may allow the use of other procedures such as manipulation and exercise. In addition, the warming effect of therapeutic ultrasound may facilitate stretching of fibrous tissue that develops as a result of prolonged inflammation. Ultrasound, therefore, is not THE treatment; rather, it is a component of the overall treatment.

Active Modalities

Following an injury, most patients move steadily through the early phases of healing and recovery. As the patient passes through the various stages of care, the body improves and the goals for treatment change. As swelling and inflammation begin to dissipate, the need for support and stabilization is replaced with a need to increase the range of motion. As pain subsides, the need for pain-relieving modalities diminishes. Attention can thus be directed at healing tissue and restoring normal function. While relief of pain and discomfort is of paramount importance to the patient, particularly in the early phases of care, restoration of normal function ultimately is the more important aspect of therapy. With improved function should come a reduction in pain and pain-associated behavior.

The changes in the patient's condition bring a simultaneous need to change the methods of treatment and the goals for care. Passive modalities should be gradually withdrawn and replaced with procedures in which the patient plays a more active role. For obvious reasons this transition may be made earlier and more completely in some patients than in others. For all practical purposes, the earlier this transition from passive care to active participation can be made, the better the prognosis and more positive the overall outcome.

The goals for the active modalities and for this phase of care include:

- improving muscle strength (*e.g.*, isometric, isotonic, isokinetic exercises)
- improving muscular and cardiovascular endurance (*e.g.*, strength training, aerobic exercises)
- improving flexibility (*e.g.*, stretching exercises)
- improving balance and coordination (*e.g.*, rocker board, gymnastic balls)
- promoting relaxation (*e.g.*, relaxation techniques, stress management)
- education of the patient (*e.g.*, back school)

Treatment Process

The primary goal of any form of therapy, whether it be manipulation, medication, electrotherapy, heat and cold, and so forth, is ***to stimulate the body to perform a specific function***. In order to select the most appropriate form of therapy, it is imperative that the clinician recognize the particular physiologic needs of the patient's condition and understand the principles of treatment as they apply to such a condition. In addition, the clinician must appreciate the psychological and emotional needs and makeup of the individual patient to be treated. Consideration must also be given to the contraindications for treatment and to patient safety. Finally, in the changing health care environment, clinicians must consider the cost effectiveness of various treatment procedures.

The treatment process itself, the body's reaction to injury (both short- and long-term), pain and pain mechanisms, and the impact of the dysfunction that develops in the locomotor system are discussed in this section. Throughout this text, therapy is discussed as it applies to the condition at hand. Treatment procedures and protocols are presented in a practical manner with attention given to methods that have been found useful in clinical practice. It may be helpful to point out that the treatment protocols and parameters presented in this text are not meant to be absolutes. Rather, they should serve as guidelines that can be modified according to the patient's particular needs and concerns.

Patient Presentation

Clear Clinical Picture

Patients present to the doctor with myriad problems and a variety of conditions, both physical and emotional. Some patients present with problems and conditions that are easily identified and provide the doctor with a clear clinical picture. For instance, the patient with a relatively minor ankle sprain does not require any particular diagnostic acumen on the part of the doctor. Diagnosis is easy and treatment procedures are uncomplicated. Treatment for this patient is usually successful and recovery is quick and complete.

Obvious Signs and Symptoms

Other patients present with problems that may not be as easily identified. The patient with a more severe injury may present with so much inflammation and pain that a complete examination may be difficult to perform. As an example, the clinician presented with a patient suffering from an acute episode of lower back pain may be unsure whether the facet joints, the intervertebral disc, or the muscles are the source of pain. The physical and orthopedic tests that ordinarily provide useful information may all be positive owing to the degree of pain and swelling. Consequently, a clear clinical picture may not readily emerge and diagnosis may challenge the clinician. Initial treatment may require attention directed at the signs and symptoms. As the condition improves in response to therapy, however, a clearer picture usually develops and a specific diagnosis determined.

Problem Behind the Problem

Still other patients present with a primary complaint that is only the "tip of the iceberg." In such a patient, there may be a variety of other conditions that are more serious and threatening. Some of these may be hidden by the magnitude of the primary complaint. Some patients, such as those with underlying substance abuse or psychological overlays, may actually attempt to hide certain components of their condition from the physician. For example, the low back pain patient who also suffers from an underlying abdominal tumor or the malingering patient who is more interested in a financial settlement than a clinical remedy.

Patients in this group represent a most difficult and sometimes perplexing clinical situation. Various treatment methods may be attempted with only limited success. When faced with an unresponsive patient, the clinician is challenged to discover the reason for the lack of improvement. Is it due to an inaccurate assessment of the patient's condition, to an inappropriate selection of treatment modalities, to a lack of compliance on the part of the patient, or perhaps to a combination of these factors? Treatment may need to be modified several times to determine the best method of managing the patient's condition.

Treatment Selection

The choice of which treatment is most appropriate for any given condition varies from patient to patient. Therapy that is effective for one patient may not necessarily be helpful for another who is suffering from a similar disorder. Likewise, the choice of which treatment to use for a given patient varies from clinician to clinician. The general practitioner confronted with a patient who is suffering from an acute episode of low back pain may prescribe moist heat, bed rest, and some form of pain relievers or muscle relaxants. The same patient presenting to a chiropractor undoubtedly will get very different care.

Even within the same specialty, the type of care a patient receives can be very different from one doctor to another. One only has to look at the seemingly endless variations and techniques in the chiropractic profession to appreciate this fact. One doctor may use an "activator," a second may use "flexion-distraction," and still another may use a "knee-chest table." Saunders (Saunders, 1985) claims that doctors tend to select treatment based largely on their individual training and philosophy rather than what is necessarily best for the patient.

From the early days of the chiropractic profession chiropractors have been trained to focus more on the cause of the condition than on the obvious signs and symptoms with which the patient presents. However, when confronted with a patient in such acute pain that an accurate assessment of the underlying nature of the condition is not readily apparent, the doctor may be forced to direct attention to the symptoms at hand. These may be pain, muscle spasm, swelling, limited range of motion, and so forth. As treatment progresses and the initial stage begins to subside, a more accurate picture of the condition may appear. Therapy can then be directed at the causative and/or contributing factors.

Treatment should be based on an objective assessment of the patient that takes into account the following factors:

Characteristics and Natural History of the Condition

For the patient with an acute episode of low back pain, the prognosis is typically quite good. Approximately 50% of these patients recover quickly within 1 week and 90% improve within the first 3 months. Consequently, aggressive or radical forms of therapy should not be necessary. However, recovery is not usually as rapid or complete for the patient with low back and leg pain. Therefore, therapy may need to be more aggressive for these patients. In addition, treatment may need to be prolonged and include efforts to rehabilitate the patient. The prognosis for the patient presenting with low back pain that is due to advanced central stenosis is clearly not optimistic. Full recovery may not be anticipated in this patient and treatment efforts may need to be directed at providing some pain and symptom relief rather than at resolving the problem. It is important to emphasize that it may not always be possible to achieve a complete resolution of the problem for each patient. Some residual pain and dysfunction may be expected and accepted.

Clinical Considerations

The otherwise healthy young adult who presents with an acute episode of low back pain often responds to a variety of physically aggressive treatment methods including the use of high-velocity manipulation (*i.e.*, the chiropractic adjustment). In contrast, the geriatric low back pain patient who presents with advanced osteoporosis obviously cannot be treated with aggressive or vigorous manual procedures. Certain treatment tools, such as traction, should be used with caution or not at all in these patients. Underlying physical problems must be taken into account when determining which treatment tools are to be used.

Treatment Considerations and Methods

When developing a therapeutic plan of action, thought must be given to the nature of the treatment itself. Treatment that is physically demanding or that places excessive financial demands on patients may not be in their best interest. It is important to consider what is planned from the perspective of all concerned. As an example, one patient seen by this author presented with neck and arm pain resulting from a herniated cervical disc. During the course of eliciting a history, the patient stated: "I can accept the pain that I have but I cannot cope with the idea of it getting worse and I have two requests of you, Doctor. First, don't make it any worse and second, don't pop my neck." Obviously, the patient's request must be respected and any high velocity manipulation should not be considered for this patient.

Treatment Goals and Plan of Care

Whenever a clinician attempts to establish a treatment plan, attempts must be made to set reasonable and attainable therapeutic goals for the patient. If treatment is to be effective, the patient and the clinician must agree on the goals and the process involved in achieving them. Patients should understand what treatment entails and what outcome to anticipate. It is necessary to develop a clear therapeutic plan of action. As treatment ensues, the plan should be evaluated and modified accordingly.

Indications and Contraindications

Each treatment procedure may be used more effectively and safely in some patients than in others. One of the factors that must be stressed is the presence of specific indications for the treatment. In addition, any factors that either contraindicate a specific treatment or call for precautions when applying treatment must be recognized. These may be divided into the following categories:

- indications—those factors that specifically indicate the application of a particular modality; for example, acute swelling is an indication for ice.
- general contraindications—include a variety of relatively common conditions in which the use of certain modalities may be unwise; for instance, diabetes and pregnancy. Each of these conditions adds elements that complicate the treatment process and, at the very least, call for additional precautions when treatment is applied.
- absolute contraindications—some treatments should absolutely not be attempted in the presence of these factors; for instance the use of shortwave diathermy in a pregnant patient in which the risk of harm to the fetus outweighs any potential benefit to the mother.

The following examples illustrate this process of developing a rational and reasonable treatment plan. Each of the cases represents a patient with a fracture. The physiologic processes, therefore, are similar. Although the ultimate treatment goals are similar (*i.e.*, to return each patient to a fully functioning, preinjury status), the methods and procedures are significantly different.

Case 1: Patient Management

Jim M., a 40-year-old, athletic male presents immediately after injuring his foot and ankle in a volleyball game. He states that he leaped in the air to strike the ball and, when he landed, he lost his footing and his ankle went out from under him. He heard a crack and feels he may have broken a bone in his foot. Evaluation of his foot demonstrates significant swelling and pain. The degree of swelling and pain inhibits attempts to evaluate the injury adequately. X-rays reveal a shaft fracture of the fifth metatarsal. In addition, you suspect that Jim has torn several ligaments in the ankle, although it is difficult at this time to determine the extent of the injury. Jim is referred to a local orthopedist for casting.

Two days after seeing Jim, he returns to your office. His foot and ankle are in a cast that extends to the midcalf. The cast is to be worn for the next 2 weeks, at which time a semirigid removable cast will be provided. Jim was provided with crutches by the orthopedist but is not using them. He feels they are cumbersome and awkward. Jim realizes that it will take time to recover but is concerned that he will lose his cardiovascular reserve and that his muscles will begin to atrophy. He asks if there is anything that he might do to minimize the impact of the immobilization. He states that he is not in any particular pain at the time and he continues his work as a teacher.

Characteristics and Natural History of the Condition

Although fractures of the fifth metatarsal usually heal within 6 to 8 weeks with little or no residual problems, the ligamentous injury to the ankle may often lead to ankle weakness and instability.

Clinical Considerations

A period of immobilization is necessary to stabilize the fracture during the early phases of healing but the resulting loss of movement comes with a price. During the time that the limb is immobilized, fibrous tissue and adhesions may develop in the joints and ligaments of the foot and ankle. These must be addressed after the cast is removed. Because the patient is not complaining of pain, pain control techniques are not necessary.

Treatment Considerations (Summary of Problems)

Swelling. Immediately after the injury swelling was significant. Once the patient was placed in a cast, however, swelling was not much of a problem. Some swelling could be expected during the course of the day, especially when the patient was on his feet.

Pain. In this instance, pain is not a particular problem. The patient may expect to experience some throbbing at night or following periods of walking or activity. Some pain may be anticipated after removal of the cast and reintroduction of activities.

Concern for Loss of Stamina and Strength. The patient expresses concern both for anticipated loss of cardiovascular reserve and for potential atrophy in the muscles of the leg.

Treatment Goals and Plan of Care

Short-Term Goals

Swelling. When the patient first presented he had significant swelling. This was treated with ice and elevation. Once the swelling had been reduced, the foot was placed in a cast. Further applications of ice are obviously not possible until the cast is removed. During the course of the day the patient may expect some swelling to occur. This may be treated with periodic elevation of the leg throughout the day. In addition, isometric contractions of the muscles in the leg may help to reduce edema. If needed, an electrical stimulator may be used to produce alternating contractions of the dorsi flexors and plantar flexors of the foot and ankle. This may provide relief from edema while the foot is in the cast.

Pain. Pain was not a particular concern for this patient. If pain had been a factor, use of a TENS device may have provided relief during the first few days.

Concern for Loss of Stamina and Strength. The patient may be given instructions to use a stationary bicycle or an upper body exerciser (hand bicycle) for a few weeks until the cast is removed. In addition, he can exercise the leg muscles by performing leg raises and hamstring curls (the cast will act as a weight).

Intermediate Goals

Swelling. Once the cast is removed and the patient begins to return to normal activities, some swelling may be anticipated, especially if he is overly aggressive with his activity level. This may now be addressed with short applications of ice and elevation.

Pain. Although pain is not a major concern in this patient, some pain may be anticipated with a return to activity. Pain control techniques probably will not be necessary unless the patient reinjures the foot and ankle.

Restoration of Function. Once the cast is removed, the primary concern should change to gradually and progressively restoring normal function and activities. The patient may begin restoring range of motion by using a rocker board in a non-weightbearing position, then progressing to an assisted and finally to a full weightbearing position. Continued use of the stationary bicycle should be encouraged. Mobilization and manipulation techniques should be helpful to assist the return to normal function.

Case 2: Patient Management

Carl F., a 22-year-old active male, presents in your office complaining of wrist pain and stiffness. Carl relates that he fractured his wrist in a skateboarding accident approximately 3 months ago. He was initially seen in a local emergency room and referred to an orthopedist. The fracture was treated with a closed reduction and he was placed in a full arm cast for 4 weeks, at which time a forearm cast was applied. On returning to the orthopedist at 6 weeks postinjury, the cast was removed and Carl was given instructions to exercise the wrist using a tennis ball and silly putty. No further appointments were made with the orthopedist.

Examination reveals significant limitation of range of motion of the wrist. Both flexion and extension are limited to approximately 50% of normal; supination and pronation are only 30% of normal. All movements are accompanied by pain at the end of range of motion. Muscle strength in the hand, wrist, and forearm is reduced. Some swelling is still present.

Characteristics and Natural History of the Condition

Unlike the previous case, fractures of the wrist often heal with significant residual problems, particularly stiffness, pain with activity, and an overall reduction in range of motion and strength. Of particular concern is the increased risk of carpal tunnel syndrome, a condition that often develops after trauma to the wrist.

Clinical Considerations

The long period of immobilization that is necessary to stabilize the fracture comes with a significant price. During the time that the hand and wrist are immobilized, fibrous tissue and adhesions may have developed in the joints and ligaments. Because the immobilization period is long with this type of fracture, the resulting adhesions become a primary problem. Restoration of normal function will take a concerted effort on the part of both the patient and the clinician.

Treatment Considerations (Summary of Problems)

Swelling. Residual swelling is often due to lack of function and to the invasion of scar tissue and adhesions.

Pain. Pain accompanies movement and patients may often avoid movement to maintain a pain-free status.

Scar Tissue and Adhesions. The deposition of scar tissue is probably the most important problem in this patient.

Loss of Range of Motion and Strength. Much of the loss in this area is a result of immobility and disuse. In addition, however, the presence of scar tissue and adhesions prevents full function.

Treatment Goals and Care Plan

Swelling. Initially, it may be helpful to attempt to reduce any swelling with a passive modality such as pulsed ultrasound. Early attempts to move the wrist may be accompanied by a temporary increase in swelling that can be treated with ice.

Pain. Because pain accompanies movement, it is important that the patient understands the need to "work through the pain." Unless the tissue is taken to the point of pain and slightly past, improvement will not be achieved.

Scar Tissue and Adhesions. Efforts to improve function will be compromised by the build-up of scar tissue and adhesions. The use of continuous ultrasound is helpful to warm these tissues prior to activity. As an alternative to ultrasound, the use of a paraffin bath may be helpful, especially for home care.

Loss of Range of Motion and Strength. Following the use of passive modalities such as ultrasound and paraffin baths, while the tissue is warm and pliable, range-of-motion exercises, passive stretching, mobilization, and manipulation will be more effective. The rocker board is a particularly helpful tool for improving the range of motion of the hand and wrist (Figure 1.1). The patient should also be given a series of exercises that he should perform daily.

These two cases provide examples of patients presenting with similar problems but who require very different treatment protocols. The method, duration, and goals for treatment vary owing to a number of the factors cited. The patient in Case 1 will heal quickly with little if any residual problems. His treatment focused on restoring normal function from the beginning with little attention directed at pain control or symptomatic relief. In contrast, the patient in Case 2 required a much more extensive treatment regimen to maximize his recovery. Although early treatment methods may be directed at controlling pain and edema, attention must shift to re-establishing range of motion, muscle strength, and coordination in all of the joints and muscles affected.

Informed Consent

In addition to clinical considerations, each patient has the right to **informed consent** prior to the initiation of any examination or treatment procedure. The patient should be informed of the following:

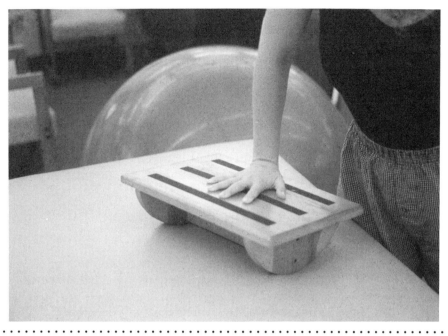

FIGURE 1.1   The rocker board is a useful tool for early rehabilitation procedures.

1. Diagnosis

2. Nature and purpose of the proposed treatment

3. Known risks and consequences of the proposed treatment excluding those eventualities that are too remote and improbable to bear significantly on the decision process of a reasonable person or are too well known to require statement

4. Benefits to be expected from the proposed treatment, with an assessment of the likelihood that the benefits can be realized

5. All alternative treatments that might reasonably be used, including all the information provided above which must be given for the alternatives as well

6. Prognosis if no treatment is given

7. All costs, including the amount and duration of pain generally involved, the potential impact on lifestyle and ability to resume work, and the economic costs of both the treatment and aftercare. The patient should be told if insurance will cover the bills (Garrett, Baillie, Garrett, 1993).

Note: At the beginning of treatment for each patient, it is helpful to inform patients of treatment goals. In describing these goals to the patient I have found it helpful to state the primary goals in the following manner: "We have three primary goals for you. First, we want to get you out of pain as quickly as we can. Second, it is important that we address the underlying problems that led to the pain, and, third, we want to teach you how to take care of yourself so that problems do not return." Initially, when patients are in pain, all of our attention will be directed at their pain and this should be communicated to the patient. Typically, some pain relief is seen relatively quickly. When patients feel some improvement we remind them of the three goals and the importance of following through until recovery is complete.

Treatment Options

It is worth noting that for any given symptom or condition there are often several effective treatment options. As stated above, the choice of treatment often is based on the personal bias of the clinician. Other factors influencing treatment options include patient preference, availability of equipment, and cost. Listed below are common symptoms and various treatment tools that can be used for them.

1. Pain and muscle guarding
   - TENS, ice, moist heat, traction, massage (passive)
   - mobilization and manipulation (passive)
2. Stiffness following inactivity
   - patient education (active)
   - exercise (active)
   - increase active range of motion with mobilization and manipulation techniques (passive)
3. Pain with mechanical stress or excessive activity
   - ice, TENS (passive)
   - supportive equipment to minimize stress or to correct faulty biomechanics (passive)
   - increase strength in supportive muscles (active)
   - alternate activity with periods of rest (passive)
4. Limitation of motion as the condition advances
   - various forms of heat (passive)
   - selective stretching techniques (active)
   - joint mobilization and manipulation techniques (passive)

5. Pain at rest in the advanced stage
   - pain-relieving modalities (passive)
   - exercise (active)
   - alternate activity with periods of rest (passive)
6. Potential deformity
   - patient education (active)
   - exercise (active)

The management of each patient should follow a logical and proven sequence that incorporates both passive and active modalities. Selection of treatment methods and procedures should be based on a variety of factors including (1) the condition at hand, (2) the individual patient, and (3) the expertise of the clinician. Goals should be identified for both the doctor and the patient. As one goal is attained, new goals should be identified and therapy modified as needed. If goals are not reached within a reasonable time period, the entire patient interaction should be reevaluated.

Reaction to Injury

Inflammatory Process

The body's reaction to trauma is consistent from injury to injury and from individual to individual. When vascularized tissue is injured, it reacts through a process known as **inflammation.** The purpose of this reaction is to control the effects of the injury and to begin the process of restoring the tissue to its normal functional state. In most instances the inflammatory process is a normal part of the body's reaction and is necessary for survival. In certain instances, however, the inflammatory process may become too aggressive or prolonged and may actually add to the problems. One only has to see a patient with an acutely sprained ankle that is swollen to several times its normal size to appreciate this fact. In such an instance much of the pain and disability may be due to the swelling rather than the injury itself. In still other conditions, such as rheumatoid arthritis, the inflammatory process is actually a part of the disease itself.

The **"cardinal signs"** of inflammation are (**SHARP**):

1. Swelling
2. Heat
3. Altered function
4. Redness
5. Pain

The inflammatory process involves two distinct series of events: (1) those involving the circulation in the injured area (**hemodynamic events**) and (2) changes in the activity of cells at various levels (**cellular events**).

Hemodynamic Events

The inflammatory process begins whenever tissue is injured and follows a predictable course (Figure 1.2). The sequence of events includes:

- an initial **vasoconstriction** of arterioles occurs that lasts only a few seconds, followed immediately by **vasodilation.**
- with vasodilation comes an increase in the amount of blood in the injured area and a rise in the intercapillary pressure.
- slight changes in the permeability of the capillary wall occur, allowing water and electrolytes (**transudate**) to escape into the extravascular area (**edema fluid**).

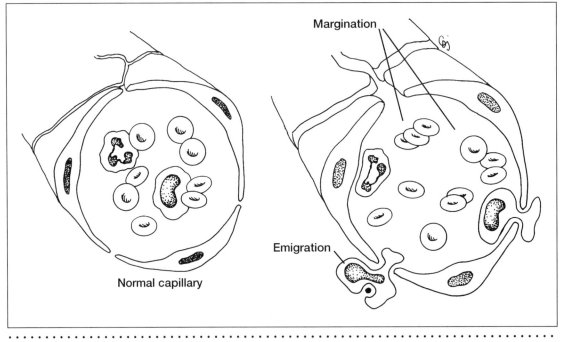

FIGURE 1.2   Inflammatory process involves a series of cellular changes.

- with increasing fluid volume in the vessels, the blood cells slow their rate of movement and align themselves along the capillary walls (**margination**).
- with increasing changes in the permeability of the capillary walls, the white blood cells begin to migrate through the walls into the surrounding tissues (**emigration**).
- the edema fluid that was initially clear now becomes viscous and cloudy (**exudate**).

Cellular Events

In addition to the changes in local circulation, there is a concomitant change in the activities of various cells in the area of the injury:

- tissue spaces and lymph vessels in the area are sealed off by the development of **fibrinogen** clots.
- **leukocytes** collect along the margin of the capillary walls.
- **monocytes** emigrate from the capillary into the surrounding tissue and change into **macrophages**, which are able to engulf debris from the injured area.
- **neutrophils** leave the blood stream and assist in the phagocytosis of debris; they contain **proteolytic enzymes** known as **lysozymes** that function to digest engulfed debris; some of the lysozymes are released into the tissue and may actually serve as an irritant that perpetuates the inflammatory reaction.

Mediators

Many of the physiologic processes described are initiated and controlled by chemicals that are released in the injured tissue (mediators). Many different chemicals that are released in the injured area serve to guide the sequence of events during the inflammatory process. Some of the more important ones are:

- **norepinephrine** causes vasoconstriction of blood vessels.
- **histamine, bradykinin, and prostaglandin** cause vasodilation.
- **complement system**, which consists of a series of proteins that participate in various stages of the inflammatory process.
- **bradykinin, serotonin, prostaglandin, and substance P** produce pain.

Healing and Repair Process

The body typically passes through the early steps of the inflammatory process in a fairly rapid sequence. It then begins the process of healing and repair. Repair occurs gradually over a period of time and sometimes is complete, although at other times it is less than perfect. Two types of cells participate in the repair process: (1) the characteristic cells of the injured area and (2) the connective tissue cells. Individual tissues vary markedly in their ability to recover. There is some evidence that the signal that triggers the body's healing response may be electrical (Becker, Selden, 1985). There is increasing interest in modalities directed at stimulating the healing process (*e.g.*, microamperage stimulation devices, electrical stimulation, ultrasound).

Characteristic Cells

When an injury occurs, the body attempts to replace any injured parts with tissue similar to the original. In some areas, such as the skin or bone, this replacement process is nearly complete and it may be difficult to distinguish the replacement tissue from the original. However, in other areas, such as articular cartilage, replacement is not always complete. In these areas, injured tissue may be replaced with a less specialized form of tissue (*i.e.*, scars and adhesions), resulting in functional changes of the injured part.

To facilitate healing and encourage the development of normal cells, it is essential that an appropriate demand be placed on injured tissue. Otherwise, injured cells may be replaced by extensive scar tissue that reduces functional integrity and may lead to chronic problems. An excellent example of the variable response of injured tissue is provided by the continuous passive movement apparatus. Salter et al. have clearly demonstrated that when articular cartilage is injured, it will heal properly only if movement is introduced during the healing stage. Without movement, the articular cartilage degenerates predictably. In the presence of movement, however, healing is rapid and may be complete (Salter et al, 1980).

Connective Tissue

During the healing process the **fibroblasts** of the surrounding connective tissue are important in sealing off the injured area and replacing damaged tissue. The fibroblasts growing in the injured area produce **collagen**. This collagen later contracts and produces a **scar**. As the healing tissue matures the scar contracts further and may eventually prevent a full return to normal function. In some instances, the scar tissue actually becomes a primary source of pain and dysfunction. The process of scar tissue formation (**fibrosis and adhesions**) is increased by immobilization and by lack of activity following an injury and is impeded by activity and movement.

Factors that Influence Inflammation and Repair

Although the process of inflammation and repair is predictable from one person to another, effectiveness and ultimate outcome are variable. Many factors influence the outcome including:

- age of the patient—typically, young persons heal faster and more completely than do older individuals.
- nutritional status—healing may be delayed or incomplete in persons who are nutritionally deficient or poorly nourished.
- poor circulation—individuals who are anemic or have poor peripheral circulation may not heal as readily (*e.g.*, diabetics).
- medication—many medications delay or prevent recovery from injury.
- the extent, type, and location of the injury.
- stress—many individuals exposed to prolonged or excessive stress may experience difficulty healing when injured.
- emotional status—some patients may not expect to recover from their injuries; others may not want to improve.

Stages of Injury

Three stages typically describe the reaction to any musculoskeletal injury: (1) the **acute** stage, (2) the **subacute** stage, and (3) the **chronic** stage. Each stage has characteristics that represent the nature of the particular physiologic processes that are involved at the time. The body's reaction to injury proceeds in a predictable manner and the passage from one stage to the next typically follows a similar time frame and sequence of events. In fact, the length of time that has elapsed since the injury occurred is one of the most common methods of determining which stage the patient is in.

Acute Stage

The acute stage is defined as that period immediately following the injury. Symptoms are usually most severe in this stage. This period has a relatively short course that typically lasts from 48 to 72 hours, although some patients may remain in this stage for a week or more. The primary characteristic during this stage is inflammation (SHARP) and it may be considered a period of "damage control." The body's resources are directed at controlling the effects of the injury and sealing off the wounded part. One of the clinical characteristics is the presence of pain in the early part of the range of motion. In some patients, even the slightest movement may produce pain. Treatment efforts are largely directed at pain relief, controlling swelling, and supporting or protecting injured tissues. Patient compliance is usually fairly good during this stage. Treatment should be combined with efforts to reassure the patient.

Subacute Stage

After passing quickly through the acute stage the body changes directions from a physiologic point of view. Attention is no longer directed at controlling the impact of the injury. Rather, the body attempts to turn its attention and resources to the task of healing and repair. This subacute period has a variable time frame that may last for several weeks. There is a gradual reduction in pain and inflammation. In addition, there is a gradually increasing degree of pain-free motion, with pain present near the end of range of motion. Patients may expect to improve 5% to 10% each day. Because many patients are still in pain during this phase, this increase in function may be used as a reasonable guideline to monitor progress.

The primary characteristic of the subacute stage is the presence of fragile, easily re-injured tissue. As the pain and symptoms subside during the subacute period, it is not uncommon to see patients exceed their functional limitations and exacerbate their condition. If this happens, the patient may re-enter the acute phase. Some patients may vacillate several times between these stages. As a patient begins to feel better, compliance tends to deteriorate. Patients often need guidance and encouragement to assist them in this phase and should be reminded of the need for functional recovery.

Chronic Stage

In some patients, recovery is delayed or incomplete and they enter the chronic stage. By their very nature, these conditions are long-lasting and may last for several months or even years. Although clinicians may not agree on when a particular problem enters the chronic stage, it is usually agreed that a condition that is not showing continued signs of improvement at 6 to 7 weeks should be considered chronic. The primary characteristic is shortened connective tissue in the form of fibrosis and adhesions. Pain is present at the end of range of motion, although the total range may be reduced.

Note: It is important to distinguish between a chronic condition and chronic pain. Chronic pain usually is described as pain that has been present for 6 months or longer (chronic pain will be discussed later in this text). Most patients with chronic problems do not have chronic pain. Instead, they often experience pain during or following certain activities and many learn to control pain and symptoms by changing their lifestyle. It is often the functional limitations that are the primary problem, not the pain.

Remodeling Stage

In addition to the three stages described above, recent attention has been directed at a fourth stage, **the remodeling stage.** As described, following an injury the body goes quickly through the acute and subacute stages. If the injury is not too severe and the treatment is appropriate, the problem heals and the condition never reaches the chronic stage. Under less than ideal circumstances, however, tissue healing may be inadequate and chronic problems may develop.

During the remodeling stage, the body attempts to return to normal structure and function. The body responds to the demand placed on it **(specific adaptation to imposed demand [SAID])** and if the demand is sufficient the injury heals with no residual defects or problems. If the demand is not appropriate, if the injury is too severe, or if the treatment is inadequate there may be residual (chronic) deficits. While there is not much reference to this stage in the literature, it remains a most important aspect of patient care and management and should be taken seriously by both the clinician and the patient. There is some evidence that this stage may last as long as 1 to 2 years post trauma in some patients.

It is important to point out that, although the remodeling stage may be lengthy, this should not be considered as an excuse for unnecessary or prolonged care. The clinician should be prepared to justify treatment during this phase of patient care. In addition, it is important that as the patient progresses he or she plays a more active role in recovery. Passive modalities should be gradually discontinued and the patient should be encouraged to exercise and return to functional activities.

Functional Restoration—the Ultimate Goal of the Chiropractor

The ultimate goal of the chiropractor is to return the injured patient to an active and productive life. Ideally, this will include eliminating both pain and the problems leading to it. When full recovery is not possible, patients must learn to manage their conditions and maintain as active a status as possible. Long periods of inactivity are both physically and psychologically detrimental to this process and may contribute to the development of chronic problems and chronic pain. Functional restoration addresses the deconditioning syndrome commonly seen in chronic pain patients. **The key to functional restoration is understanding that teaching and training patients what to do for themselves is the goal of chronic pain management.** Passive intervention may be a catalyst for this process, but **the focus of care must be on promotion of patient independence** during functional restoration. Although the concepts of functional restoration are often reserved for the chronic pain patient, a similar approach that employs active therapy with supportive use of passive modalities is helpful for all patients. Patients should not be allowed to become dependent on treatment. Rather, they should be encouraged to recover.

The concept of functional restoration includes:

- assessment of physical capacity.
- guided rehabilitation procedures.
- measurement of outcomes.

Relationship Between Pain and Pathology

Although most patients presenting to a chiropractor recover quickly, a small percentage of individuals do not improve. Some may continue to have problems long after the presenting condition has been treated. A small number of patients develop chronic problems that linger for years. It is important to recognize that the relationship between the severity of the presenting condition and the degree of pain and other symptoms that a patient experiences is not consistent from one patient to another. It should also be appreciated that the degree of pain and symptoms experienced by the patient may not correlate to the degree of pathology that is present.

If we use the patient with back pain as an example, it is evident that the relationship between spinal pathology and the presence of back pain is not clearly established. Many patients with severe pathology have very few symptoms. On the other hand, patients with severe symptoms may have little or no definitive pathology. The evidence indicates that many of the factors that may be positively associated with back pain, especially those associated with chronic or disabling back pain, are psychosocial. They include problems such as:

- job and life satisfaction
- secondary gain
- greater frequency of neurosis, migraine, ulcer
- alcohol and tobacco use

With these things in mind, it is important that the clinician take steps to enable patients to participate in their own recovery. Patients who are allowed to linger indefinitely on passive modalities may become dependent on the clinician and the treatment. In contrast, patients who are encouraged to take control of their situation and who are placed in active therapy programs tend to recover more quickly and more completely.

Deconditioning Syndrome

The patient who has been disabled by pain, such as chronic back pain, for a prolonged period of time often becomes less and less active. This individual may or may not be working. With a reduction in activity comes changes such as:

- weight gain
- loss of muscle strength and endurance
- loss of cardiovascular endurance
- loss of balance and coordination
- joint stiffness
- muscle tightness
- depression

An athlete who is injured seriously usually goes through an extended period of rehabilitation prior to resuming normal activities. Until recently, the back-injured individual was not considered a candidate for similar rehabilitation. Mayer et al (Mayer, Mooney, Gatchel, 1991) introduced the concept of "functional restoration" for the back-injured individual. They took a "sports medicine approach" to the problem of back pain. Others have since modified this approach to patient care in an effort to restore the nonathlete to preinjury status and activities.

Rehabilitation of the Chronic Pain Patient

Functional restoration, along with patient education and psychosocial support, are the main features of a rehabilitation program for patients with chronic problems. Functional restoration occurs in three stages: (1) patient reactivation, (2) progressive physical training, and (3) activity or work hardening (Liebensohn, 1991).

Functional Capacity Assessment

Evaluation of a recovering patient should involve two parts: (1) the classic orthopedic/neurologic examination to attempt to identify the pathology and (2) the functional capacity assessment, which should include both qualitative and quantitative components.

Baseline Tests of Functional Capacity

- evaluation of muscle strength
- muscle endurance or muscular fatigue
- movement coordination
- mobility and flexibility
- poor balance and coordination
- cardiovascular endurance

Rehabilitation Goals

Before physical reactivation and training can begin, patients must be informed about their rehabilitation goals. Based on their functional capacity assessment, along with occupational and recreational history, realistic rehabilitation goals are mutually decided on by patient and doctor. Goal setting is a crucial step toward a successful rehabilitation outcome.

Patient Reactivation—The First Level

The first objective of training is to motivate the patient to perform repetitive movements that are safe. The initial goals during this stage are to activate the patient, increase endorphins, decrease fear of movement, explore movements, and improve cardiovascular fitness, which involves both cardiovascular training and static and dynamic exercise. Passive modalities are useful in this phase to reduce pain and swelling and facilitate a return to activity.

Upon successful reactivation of the patient, reassessment of the patient's functional capacity and training range are in order. Improvements should be recorded and communicated to the patient. New goals should be set.

Functional Restoration—The Second Level

Functional restoration is the most important part of rehabilitation of the chronic pain patient. It involves reactivating patients, guiding them through a progressive, active training regimen, and ultimately preparing them for return to their specific occupational or recreational activities. Functional capacity assessment provides the information necessary to guide patients through the necessary stages of functional restoration.

Once the patient has become reactivated and is beginning to lose fear of movement and activity, it is time to begin gradually expanding training range and increasing the demands on movements. Gradually improving mobility or flexibility, strength, endurance, coordination, and balance becomes the focus of the second phase of training. Passive modalities may provide support for patients during this phase by reducing symptoms and encouraging greater levels of activity.

Progressive resistance exercises are a classic way to improve strength and endurance of muscles. Isotonic, isokinetic, or free weight equipment, if available, can be useful for improving strength and endurance of specific movements. Both concentric and eccentric movements should be trained. Developing control and skill during training is often more important than maximizing repetitions or load. Coordination and stabilization exercises to improve efficiency and control during performance of basic movements are invaluable in training the chronic pain patient. These exercises focus on maintaining proper form and staying within the functional training range. Gymnastic balls, wall pulleys, and the rocker board are useful here (Figure 1.3).

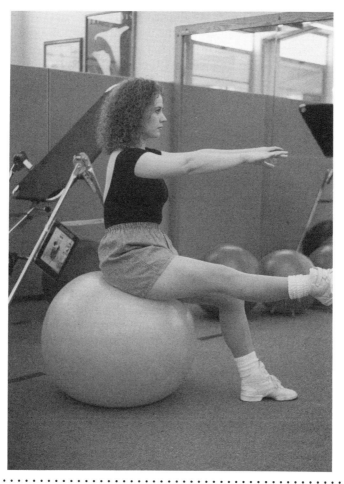

FIGURE 1.3   The gym ball is useful to improve coordination and stabilization.

Work or Activity Hardening — The Third Level

More advanced rehabilitation procedures incorporate the concepts of work-hardening and activity-specific training. This may require outside expertise (*e.g.*, an occupational therapist or vocational rehabilitation specialist). The goal of this final stage of training is to reintegrate an individual back to preinjury status or predisability role.

Summary of Functional Restoration Outcome Measures

With the changes in health care that are taking place today comes an increasing demand for **outcome measures**. Not only must modalities and procedures be clinically effective, they must also be shown to be cost effective. Clinicians must be able to document that treatment methods are accomplishing the task of returning patients to preinjury status effectively and efficiently. In addition to a reduction in pain and symptoms, some examples of outcome measures include:

- return to work
- additional surgeries
- visiting additional health care professionals
- average number of visits to health care professionals
- average percent of recurrent injuries (among those returning to work)
- unresolved Worker's Compensation litigation cases

Summary

The appropriate application of treatment procedures, combined with a unique perspective regarding the complex nature of musculoskeletal injuries, places the chiropractor in an important position in today's changing health care arena. At the time of this writing, the use of active care is becoming more established. The role for passive modalities and passive patient care procedures is declining. The purpose of this text is to allow the student of chiropractic to develop a clear and practical understanding of the important role that these passive elements play in enabling patients to become active.

References and Suggested Reading

Agency for Health Care Policy and Research. Guidelines for Acute Low Back Pain. U.S. Dept. of Health and Human Services, PHS, AHCPR Pub No. 95-0642, Rockville, MD, 1994.

Becker RO, Selden G. The body electric: electromagnetism and the foundation of life. New York: William Morrow and Co., 1985.

Garrett TM, Baillie HW, Garrett RM. Health care ethics, 2nd ed. Englewood Cliffs, NJ: Prentice Hall, 1993.

Liebensohn C. Rehabilitation. Part I: Overview. CCA Journal 1991; 16(7):25-28.

Mayer TG, Mooney V, Gatchel RJ. Contemporary conservative care for spinal disorders. Philadelphia: Lea and Febiger, 1991.

Salter RB, Simmonds DR, Malcolm BW, et al. The biological effect of continuous passive motion in healing of full thickness defects in articular cartilage. J Bone Joint Surg Am 1980; 62A(8):1232-1251.

Saunders HD. Evaluation, treatment and prevention of musculoskeletal disorders. Minneapolis: Viking Press, 1985.

Spitzer WO. Scientific approach to the assessment and management of activity-related spinal disorders. A monograph for clinicians: report of the Quebec Task Force on Spinal Disorders. Spine 1987;12(75): 56-59 (supplement).

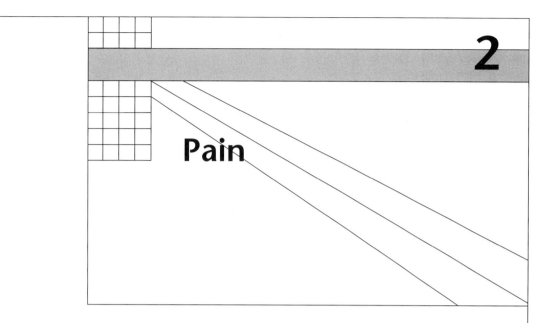

2

Pain

Learning Objectives

At the completion of this chapter, you should be able to:

1. Define pain.
2. Describe how pain is perceived and transmitted.
3. Differentiate between acute and chronic pain.
4. Describe how pain is measured:
   - Visual Analog Scale
   - pain drawing
   - McGill Pain Questionnaire
5. Describe the information concerning pain that is retrieved from patients during the case history.
6. Describe the following theories of pain modulation:
   - pain-gating mechanism
   - release of endogenous opiates
   - counterirritation
   - conduction block
   - exogenous pharmaceuticals

Pain is one of the most common reasons that an individual seeks medical care. In fact, back pain is the second leading cause for seeking the advice of a doctor. Head pain ranks as the number three reason. As such, it is important that the chiropractor understand the mechanisms by which pain is produced, the mechanics of pain perception, individual variations in the perception of and reaction to pain, methods of measuring pain, theories of pain modulation and suppression, and the treatment methods used to reduce or eliminate pain.

Pain is defined as "an unpleasant sensory and emotional experience associated with actual or potential tissue damage," or it is described in terms of such damage. The subject of pain has been studied for centuries, and volumes have been written in an attempt to understand better its complex nature. Recent investigations found answers to many questions regarding the exact mechanisms through which pain is felt, interpreted, and reduced. Currently, however, our understanding remains somewhat limited and there are more questions than answers about pain.

This chapter provides the reader with an overview of current information about pain. Specific attention is given to those methods of pain assessment and pain control that are applicable to the chiropractic practice and to the treatment of musculoskeletal conditions. A foundation for treatment must be based on: (1) a thorough knowledge of the condition, (2) the theories of pain control, and (3) the mechanisms of action of treatment modalities and techniques.

Pain Perception

For pain to be experienced, several factors must be present. First, there must be a stimulus that is unpleasant (**noxious**). Interestingly, individuals may disagree on what actually constitutes a noxious stimulus. What is painful for one patient may be only annoying to another. Second, there must be some type of receptor that is activated by the noxious stimulus. Although there may be many different types of receptors capable of responding to a noxious stimulus, **free nerve endings** are probably the best example of a pain receptor (Figure 2.1). Tissue that contains a high concentration of free nerve endings is considered pain sensitive, whereas tissue that is devoid of these receptors may be insensitive to pain. Once activated, the noxious stimulus must be transmitted to the central nervous system where it must reach a higher center that recognizes the stimulus. The sensation of pain is transmitted through nerve fibers known as nociceptors. Although it is not entirely clear how transmission occurs, there are several classic theories that explain the transmission of pain.

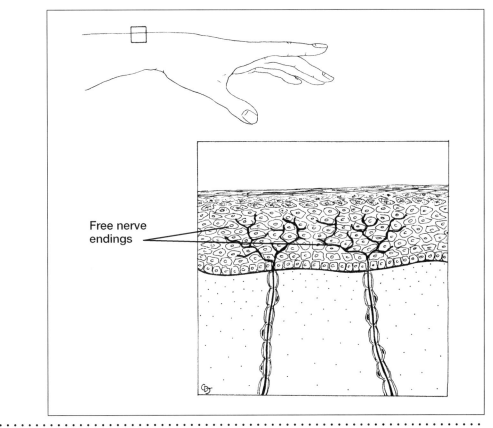

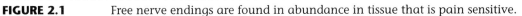

FIGURE 2.1 Free nerve endings are found in abundance in tissue that is pain sensitive.

Theories of Pain Perception

Specificity Theory

Historically, it has been known that specific nerve fibers and nerve endings are necessary for noxious stimuli to be transmitted (Figure 2.2). It has been postulated that there are four distinct classes of cutaneous sensations: warm, cold, touch, and pain, with each served by a specific receptor and neurologic pathway (von Frey, 1895, Muller, 1942). Although this theory of pain transmission is an oversimplification, components of it influence modern understanding of pain perception. First, it is clear that there are specialized somatosensory receptors that respond optimally to specific types of stimuli. Nociceptors are but one of these classes of receptors. Second, the central location of the primary afferent neurons and ascending pathways is a critical factor in distinguishing the nature of the peripheral stimulus (Price, 1988).

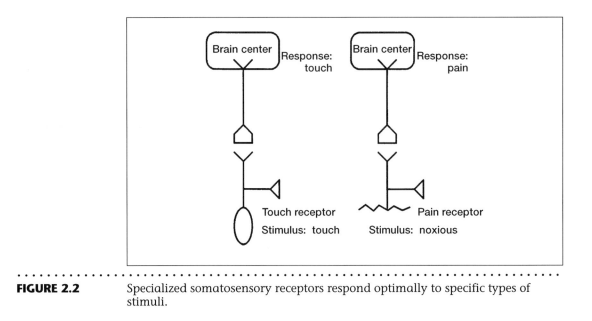

FIGURE 2.2   Specialized somatosensory receptors respond optimally to specific types of stimuli.

Pattern Theory

A second theory is based on the concept that most cutaneous receptors are morphologically similar. In addition, many free nerve endings, such as those in the cornea, respond nonselectively to mechanical, thermal, and chemical stimuli (Weddell, 1955). It has been theorized that most sensory fibers may transmit noxious impulses providing the stimulus fits a specific pattern or form (Figure 2.3). In other words, those fibers that are normally responsible for the transmission of light touch, vibration, deep touch, and temperature may send painful messages to the central nervous system if they are stimulated in a particularly intense or abnormal manner.

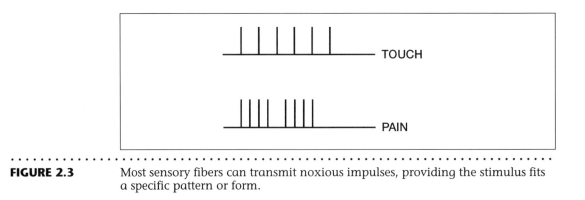

FIGURE 2.3   Most sensory fibers can transmit noxious impulses, providing the stimulus fits a specific pattern or form.

Although many primary nociceptive afferent neurons respond to more than one type of physical stimulus, there is no evidence for any type of complex impulse interval patterning. However, these neurons generally have thresholds below that which would be considered painful and they respond to increasingly painful stimulus intensities with increasing impulse frequencies, which indicates that impulse frequency is a critical factor in distinguishing noxious from non-noxious stimuli. Impulse frequency is clearly part of the overall pattern of input to ascending sensory pathways (Price, 1988).

In addition to the factors discussed above, another possibility exists. Most nociceptive primary afferents respond to more than one form of stimulation so that receptor specificity is relative and not absolute. Consequently, the composition of activated primary afferents may be different for various forms of stimulation. The overall spatial and temporal composition of neuronal activation must be an integral factor in distinguishing the type of stimulus (Price, 1988).

Summation Theory

Livingstone postulated that excessive stimulation of sensory fibers results in the transmission of noxious impulses. He stated that pathologic activation of sensory nerves, seen after peripheral nerve damage, initiated a closed self-exciting loop of neuronal activity, a kind of reverberatory circuit (Livingstone, 1943). Although there does not appear to be any anatomic basis for this circuitry, it does appear that some nociceptive afferents, especially C polymodal afferents, are likely to release long-duration neurotransmitters or neuromodulatory substances. Slow, temporal summation mechanisms, spatial recruitment mechanisms, and after-response mechanisms clearly exist within the dorsal horn.

Sensory Interaction Theory

Similar in concept to the idea of central summation is the theory that a specialized system exists to control sensory input. This system normally prevents summation from occurring. Destruction of this system results in pathologic pain states (Goldsheider, 1894). It is postulated that a rapidly conducting system inhibits synaptic transmission in a more slowly conducting nociceptive system. Under certain conditions, the fast conducting system is said to lose its inhibitory control over the slow one with resultant pain (Melzack, 1973, Melzack and Wall, 1983).

Noordenbos refined this theory. He stated that small afferents carried noxious sensations, whereas the larger afferents played an inhibitory role (Noordenbos, 1959). From this idea came the proposal that pain perception was determined by the balance of input from large and small fibers. It is now apparent that stimulation of large, fast-conducting mechanosensitive afferents does inhibit nociceptive responses (Price, 1988).

In all probability, each of these mechanisms operates individually or collectively under different circumstances. The collective interaction of neuronal activity leads to the complex system of pain perception.

Nociceptors

A full 61 years prior to their discovery, Sherrington proposed the existence of specialized receptors that were necessary to protect organisms from tissue damage. He labeled these afferent organs *nociceptors* (Sherrington, 1906). The first characterization of primary nociceptive afferent neurons appeared in the mid 1960s. Since then, considerable evidence has accumulated that a significant portion of cutaneous nerve afferents are uniquely responsive to damaging or potentially damaging stimuli.

Spinal cord neurons that respond exclusively to noxious input are found in high concentrations in the superficial layers of the dorsal horn (laminae I-II) and to a lesser extent in layers IV-V (Figure 2.4). The major sources of input to these neurons are high-threshold A delta mechanosensitive fibers, A delta heat sensitive fibers, and C polymodal afferents.

There are two types of sensory fibers that are thought to carry painful impulses to the central nervous system (CNS). The first, the **A delta fibers**, are fast, finely myelinated fibers that are rapidly accommodating. They appear to be responsible for the transmission of the sharp pain that is characteristic of many acute conditions. This pain is sometimes referred to as **first order pain**. These superficial fibers are found predominantly in the skin and in small numbers in the joints and muscles. They are sensitive to high-intensity mechanical stimuli; a small number are also sensitive to noxious temperatures.

The second fiber type, the **C fibers**, are slow, small, unmyelinated fibers that are found in the deeper layers of the skin and in virtually every other tissue except the nervous system. These fibers are sensitive to mechanical, thermal, and chemical noxious stimuli. C polymodal fibers are the free nerve endings in which the nerve terminals themselves are the receptors. They are commonly silent unless activated by noxious stimulation. Unlike the A delta fibers, the C fibers are slowly accommodating. They are thought to be responsible for the transmission of the dull, aching type of pain that is often characteristic of more chronic conditions. This is sometimes referred to as **second order pain**. The transmitter substance for these fibers is probably substance P (Wells, et al, 1988).

Acute and Chronic Pain

There is a great deal of variation in the description of pain from one patient to the next, although there is some similarity in the terms used to describe pain arising from an acute injury compared with that of a chronic nature.

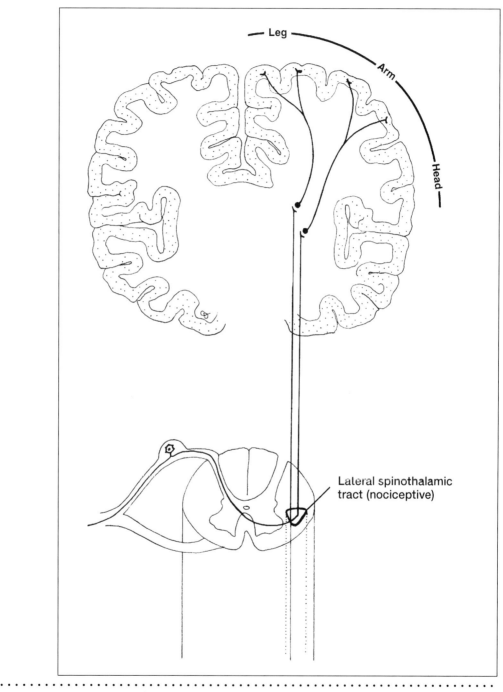

FIGURE 2.4   Transmission of painful impulses occurs via specific spinal cord tracts.

There is a similar comparison between some types of musculoskeletal pain and the deeper pain found in visceral disorders.

Acute Pain

Acute pain is described as pain arising from a recent injury. It is usually of a short duration ranging from several days to a few weeks. This type of pain is typically easily localized by the patient and appears to be superficially located. It is often described in terms of "sharp, pricking, tingling, and so forth" and is thought to be due to irritation of superficial A delta fibers.

Case Example. A patient presents complaining of an acute episode of lower back pain. When asked to locate the pain the patient bends backward and slightly to one side. He points with a finger to the middle of the lower back and states: "It hurts right there." When questioned about the quality of the pain, he describes it as "like someone is sticking an ice pick in my back."

Acute pain serves to protect the body from further injury and should not necessarily be eliminated. Rather, it should be controlled or modified to a tolerable level. Efforts to eradicate acute pain completely may lead to further injury.

Note: Frequently a patient with acute pain is given muscle relaxants. Although this may not directly affect the pain, it does calm the patient. It may be helpful to teach the patient relaxation techniques to provide similar relief.

Chronic Pain

By definition, chronic pain lasts longer and may range from several months to many years. By convention, a chronic pain is one that has persisted for a period of longer than 6 months. Chronic pain appears to be diffuse and is often difficult for the patient to locate precisely. It appears to be deeply seated and is often described in terms of "aching, burning, throbbing." It is thought to be due to activation of deeper C fibers.

Case Example. A patient presents with a back problem of several months duration. When asked to locate the source of his pain he is unable to precisely identify any specific area. Rather, he places his hand over the lower back and moves it around stating: "It hurts here." He describes the quality of his pain as being "like a toothache in my back."

Unlike acute pain, chronic pain no longer serves any useful biologic purpose. In fact, the pain itself may become the primary disease process. It is often associated with complex and significant psychological problems. Some patients learn to use the pain to their advantage (*e.g.,* easier work environment or more cooperative spouse). Others may become "addicted" to the pain. It may be associated with substance abuse (*e.g.,* drugs, alcohol). One of the currently popular medical treatments for chronic pain patients is the use of antidepressant medication.

Note: It is important to differentiate the patient with chronic pain from the patient with pain from a chronic condition. As stated in Chapter 1, a chronic condition is one that has persisted for a period of 6 to 7 weeks and is not showing continued signs of improvement. Such conditions often are accompanied by intermittent pain that comes and goes with changes in activity. Not all chronic conditions are accompanied by pain. In contrast, chronic pain, by definition, has persisted for 6 months or longer. Often, the degree of pain is difficult to correlate with the degree of pathology present or with the clinical findings.

Pain Measurement

There is tremendous variation in the degree to which individual patients perceive pain. There are also differences in the degree to which individuals react to pain and to painful stimuli. One of the most difficult problems for the clinician is determining exactly how much pain the patient actually feels, and how this pain is affected over the duration of the treatment. Efforts must be made to identify the location of any pain that the patient experiences. In addition, pain should be both quantified and qualified. How much pain is there and what is it like? How does the pain affect function and activities of daily living? Above all, it is important to establish that the pain the patient is experiencing is consistent with the clinical findings.

Patient History—OPQRST Format

One of the most important aspects of the patient history is achieving a clear description of the degree, location, and quality of the patient's pain. It is suggested that the OPQRST format be used as a guide. This format includes information on onset, provocation and palliation, quality, radiation, severity, and temporal factors.

Onset

When did the pain begin and what was the mechanism of injury? A patient who describes the onset of pain after a motor vehicle accident does not reveal much information. The patient who accurately describes the circumstances of the accident may provide valuable information. Consider the following answers to the question: "When did your pain begin?"

Patient A. "I was in a car accident several days ago and the pain began right after the accident."

Patient B. "I was involved in a car accident 3 days ago. My car was rear-ended by another vehicle that was traveling approximately 45 miles per hour. My car was pushed through an intersection and into a telephone pole. My head struck the windshield and I immediately felt a sharp pain in my neck."

Provocative and Palliative Factors

The purpose of this question is to identify those factors that make the pain worse and those factors that ease the pain.

Patient A. "My neck hurts when I move it and it feels better when I rest."

Patient B. "My neck hurts when I move it, especially when I try to turn and look over my right shoulder to back out of the driveway. It feels much better when I lie down but I find I must use a firm pillow for support."

Quality

This question is intended to gain a picture of the type of pain the patient is experiencing. It is important to allow the patient to describe the pain in his or her own words.

Patient A. "My neck hurts."

Patient B. "My neck aches most of the time, but when I move I have a sharp pain that is like an electrical shock."

Radiation

Does the pain radiate or move? If so, what activities or circumstances provoke this radiation?

Patient A. "The pain goes down my arm."

Patient B. "As the day goes on and I tire, the pain goes down my right arm. I also experience an electrical shock in my arm whenever I sneeze or cough."

Severity

How bad is the pain? It is customary to evaluate the intensity of a patient's pain using a scale from 0 to 10, with 0 being no pain and 10 being the worse imaginable pain or the worst pain the patient has experienced (see Visual Analog Scale). Patients will often reveal historical information when they compare the pain they are presently describing. It is helpful to question patients about the pain at both its greatest and its current intensity.

Patient A. "The pain is 8 out of 10."

Patient B. "The pain is now probably a 6. When I move or sneeze it increases to perhaps 7 or 8. The worst pain that I ever felt, what I would consider a 10, would be a broken bone." It would seem reasonable to assume that this patient has had a broken bone at some point in life, a fact that may or may not have been otherwise revealed in the history.

Temporal

How has the pain changed with time? Is the pain improving, decreasing, or not changing? How does the pain behave during a typical day?

Patient A. "The pain is getting worse."

Patient B. "The pain seems to be increasing. My neck hurt immediately after the accident but the last couple of days I think it is worse. My neck is stiff and sore in the morning when I first get up. After I take a shower I feel better for a little while but the pain gets progressively more intense as the day goes on."

It is easy to see that Patient B has provided a much clearer picture to the doctor. How the patient describes the pain is an important step in establishing the nature and severity of the injury. The patient's description may also provide valuable clues regarding the most appropriate treatment. For example, if a patient states that the pain is an 8 on a 0 to 10 scale, pain relief must become a primary therapeutic goal. On the other hand, if a patient describes the pain as a 3 or 4, pain relief is not so important. Treatment goals for this patient may include early restoration of function rather than focusing on pain relief.

Note: It is important to evaluate whether or not the patient's description of the pain makes sense when compared to the clinical findings. If the objective findings do not substantiate the description of pain, the clinician must attempt to determine why such a discrepancy exists. Is there something more serious that is complicating the picture? Is the patient somatising or magnifying the symptoms? Or, perhaps, is the patient malingering?

Pain Assessment Tools

Many attempts have been made to quantify and qualify pain. Some of the more common and the more useful ones are: (1) the Visual Analog Scale, (2) the Pain Drawing, and (3) the McGill Pain Questionnaire. Other pain measurement tools are described in Appendix A: Pain Measurement Tools.

Visual Analog Scale

The Visual Analog Scale (VAS) consists of a line 10 cm in length (Figure 2.5). At one end of the line is a zero and the words "**NO PAIN.**" At the other end of the line is the number 10 and the words "**WORSE PAIN IMAGINABLE.**" The patient is asked to place a mark, somewhere on the line at a point corresponding to the level of pain. The advantages of the VAS are its ease of use and its reliability in comparing pain from one visit with subsequent visits. It is **NOT** useful in comparing the pain of one patient with that of another. It should be noted that the VAS may be performed verbally by asking the patient to grade the pain on a scale of 0 to 10, with 0 being "**NO PAIN**" and

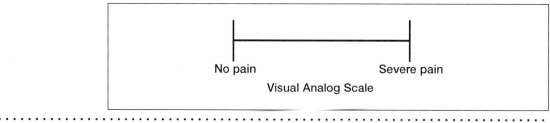

FIGURE 2.5   One version of the Visual Analog Scale consists of a line that is 10 cm long.

10 being the **"WORST IMAGINABLE PAIN."** It is suggested that a VAS be performed at the time of the first examination. Some form of VAS, either visual or verbal, should be performed once weekly during the course of treating the patient's pain.

Pain Drawing

This consists of the outline of a person seen from the front and back and from both sides (Figure 2.6). The patient is asked to mark the location of the pain on the figures provided. The characteristics of the pain (*e.g.,* sharp, tingling, stabbing, and so forth) may be indicated by providing a scale or legend with the drawing. The pain drawing is a useful tool to evaluate both the location and intensity of pain. The extent of the painful area may be monitored over time. In addition, the pain drawing may provide valuable information regarding the presence of any suspected psychological overlay (Figure 2.7). The pain drawing is useful at the time of the initial examination and may be repeated at subsequent reevaluations.

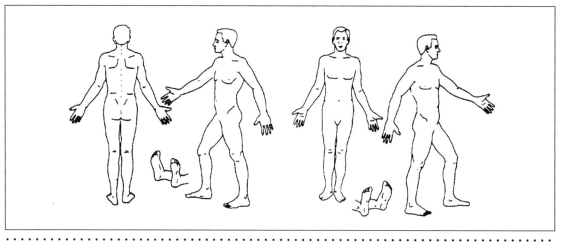

FIGURE 2.6   A pain drawing often is used to illustrate the location of pain.

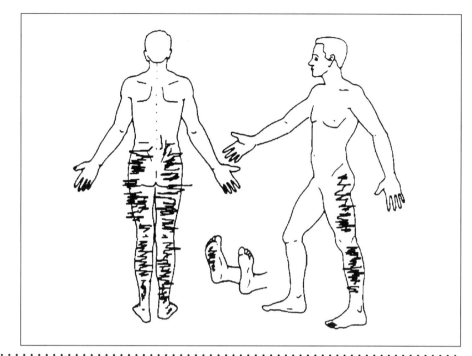

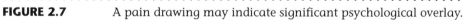

FIGURE 2.7   A pain drawing may indicate significant psychological overlay.

McGill Pain Questionnaire

There are a number of tools used to evaluate the complaint of pain. Of these, one of the most widely used is the McGill Pain Questionnaire, which consists of a sheet of paper containing 20 groups of words (Figure 2.8). The patient is asked to circle the word in each group that most closely resembles the pain. It is important that patients understand that they do not have to circle a word in each group but that they cannot circle more than one word in any group (it may be necessary to assist some patients with this form).

Word groups 1 through 11 are described as **sensory** and assess the patient's perceptions of the sensory dimension of the pain. Word groups 12 through 15 are **affective** and provide the examiner with an idea of the effect the pain has had on the patient. Word group 16 **evaluates** and measures the intensity dimension of the patient's pain. Word groups 17 through 20 are **miscellaneous** dimensions of pain perception. The descriptors in each category are ranked in terms of increasing intensity from top to bottom. The questionnaire may be scored on the basis of the number of words chosen from among the 20 category scales or according to the sum of the rank values of the descriptors chosen. It is suggested that the McGill Pain Questionnaire be used at the time of a patient's initial visit. Other pain questionnaires may be substituted (see Appendix A: Pain Measurement Instruments).

Instructions on Use
Look carefully at the twenty groups of words. If any word in any group applies to your pain, please circle that word - but do not circle more than *one word in any one group* - so you must choose the *most suitable word* in that group. In groups that do not apply to your pain, there is no need to circle *any* word - just leave them as they are.

Group 1	Group 2	Group 3	Group 4	Group 5
Flickering Quivering Pulsing Throbbing Beating	Jumping Flashing Shooting	Pricking Boring Drilling Stabbing Lancinating	Sharp Gritting Lacerating	Pinching Pressing Gnawing Cramping Crushing
Group 6	**Group 7**	**Group 8**	**Group 9**	**Group 10**
Tugging Pulling Wrenching	Hot Burning Scalding Searing	Tingling Itching Smarting Stinging	Dull Sore Hurting Aching Heavy	Tender Taut Rasping Splitting
Group 11	**Group 12**	**Group 13**	**Group 14**	**Group 15**
Tiring Exhausting	Sickening Suffocating	Fearful Frightful Terrifying	Punishing Grueling Cruel Vicious Killing	Wretched Blinding
Group 16	**Group 17**	**Group 18**	**Group 19**	**Group 20**
Annoying Troublesome Miserable Intense Unbearable	Spreading Radiating Penetrating Piercing	Tight Numb Drawing Squeezing Tearing	Cool Cold Freezing	Nagging Nauseating Agonizing Dreadful Torturing

FIGURE 2.8   The McGill Pain Questionnaire is one method of assessing the quality of pain.

Theories of Pain Modulation

Whereas the measurement and documentation of pain remains an important clinical consideration, pain relief is more important to the patient, particularly in the early phase of care. The primary application of many of the therapeutic modalities discussed in this text is directed at breaking the **"pain-spasm-pain"** cycle.

Over the years, many theories have been developed to explain how pain is modified or controlled. Some of the more popular are: (1) the gate theory of pain control, (2) the release of endogenous opiates, (3) counter-irritation, (4) the use of exogenous pharmaceuticals, and (5) nerve block (conduction block). Of these theories, the gate theory is probably best known.

Gate Theory of Pain Control

In 1965, Melzack and Wall combined features of the classic models of pain mechanisms into a unified conceptual schema that has been termed "**the gate theory of pain control**" (Melzack and Wall, 1965). They postulated that there exists a "physiologic gate" in the substantia gelatinosa of the dorsal horn of the spinal cord. This spinal gate is influenced by the relative amount of activity in the large diameter (A delta) sensory fibers and small diameter fibers. Activity in large fibers tends to inhibit transmission (close the gate), whereas an increase in small-diameter fiber activity tends to facilitate transmission (open the gate). When the gate is opened, the loss of inhibitory activity allows the patient to perceive pain; when closed, however, the sensation of pain is blocked at the cord level. Melzack and Wall stated that the gate could be closed by stimulation of the large, superficial sensory fibers (A delta). This can be achieved via the following: transcutaneous electrical nerve stimulation (TENS), massage, stroking, heat, cold, and vibration.

Since its initial introduction, the gate theory has come under considerable scrutiny. Although it is clear that the original theory is not completely accurate in all its forms, the principal tenets remain intact. A modification of the theory should include: (1) stimulation of both mechanoreceptive and nociceptive afferents can evoke inhibition, (2) not all nociceptive neurons of the dorsal horn receive input from both large and small afferents (some nociceptive-specific neurons receive input only from the latter), and (3) not all types of primary nociceptive afferents exert the same central effects. In addition to the changes to the proposed mechanism described above, it has become clear that the transmission of impulses is modulated by descending control systems as well as by local circuit interneurons.

It is fair to state that the gate theory is not an adequate explanation of pain mechanisms. Price states that the tenets of the theory are not so much incorrect as they are too general (Price, 1988). Nevertheless, Melzack and Wall exerted a significant influence on the study of pain and pain mechanisms. Their theory has served as the basis for a variety of treatment protocols (especially the use of TENS) and subsequent pain theories (Melzack, Wall, 1983).

Release of Endogenous Opiates

It has been observed that, under certain conditions, the body releases a group of chemicals that have been referred to as "naturally occurring morphinelike substances." The most well-known of these substances is beta-endorphin, which is said to be approximately 48 times the strength of morphine (others include dynorphin and enkephalin). These chemical pain suppressors are produced in the anterior lobe of the pituitary gland. They exhibit a systemic inhibitory effect and are involved in the degradation of several potent pain-producing chemicals. The production of these endorphins is enhanced by a variety of conditions, including vigorous exercise, deep relaxation, acupuncture, and low-frequency—high-intensity electrical stimulation (LoTENS). Manipulation recently has been shown to induce a mild increase in beta endorphin levels (Vernon, 1991).

Counterirritation

The counterirritation phenomena (*i.e.*, the pain-relieving effects of painful stimuli) have been known for centuries. The idea is basically, "pain inhibits pain." A common, everyday example may be used to illustrate this process. Consider the individual who is suffering from a headache. This person drops an object and fractures a toe. Temporarily at least, the headache is replaced with pain from the injured toe. Several types of counter irritants (*e.g.*, cold, heat, mechanical, and electrical) have been used with one of the most effective being the application of painful cold (*i.e.*, ice massage). Painful electrical stimulation is described as "hypalgesia by hyperstimulation," a form of counterirritant. There is some evidence that electrical acupuncture point stimulation must be as strong as the patient can tolerate for a reliable pain-relieving effect to occur.

Exogenous Pharmaceuticals

The medical profession has employed a variety of pain-suppressing chemical agents in an effort to relieve or prevent pain. Many of these chemicals, such as the nonsteroidal anti-inflammatory drugs (NSAIDs) block the inflammatory process. Others block the transmission of painful impulses by interfering with the relay of information at the synapse. Some reduce muscle tension and exert a sedating effect on the body. While producing the desired effect, many of these chemicals actually interfere with the healing process and may add to the problems if relied on too heavily.

Nerve Block (Conduction Block)

There is some evidence that high-frequency electrical stimulation may actually block the transmission of sensory stimuli. This may be similar to the muscle fatigue that is known to occur with particular applications of electrical stimulation. The frequency-dependent conduction block theory proposes that a pain-transmitting neuron can be rendered inactive or blocked by adjusting the frequency of the impulse so that it is delivered before all the ionic channels in that neuron respond. Because no action potential is generated by the neuron, pain sensation is not felt.

Summary

Although significant advances have been made in our knowledge of pain and pain mechanisms, current understanding of pain remains far from complete. As a better understanding develops other mechanisms undoubtedly will appear. With increasing knowledge may come safer and more effective methods of pain control. It is important to emphasize that most patients presenting to a chiropractor will improve quickly. As patients improve, attention should be diverted from pain to function.

References and Suggested Reading

Goldscheider, A. Ueber den Schmerz in physiologischer und klinischer. Hinsicht: Hirschwald, 1894.

Livingstone WK. Pain mechanisms. New York: Macmillan, 1943.

Melzack R, Wall PD. Pain mechanisms: a new theory. Science 1965;150:971-979.

Melzack R. The puzzle of pain. New York: Basic Books, 1973.

Melzack R, Wall PD. The challenge of pain. New York: Basic Books, 1983.

Muller J. Elements of physiology. London: Taylor, 1942.

Noordenbos W. Pain. Amsterdam: Elsevier, 1959.

Price DD. Psychological and neural mechanisms of pain. New York: Raven Press, 1988, 212-231.

Sherrington DS. The integrative action of the nervous system. New York: Scribners, 1906.

Vernon HT, Spinal manipulation and headaches of cervical origin. A review of literature and presentation of cases. J Man Med 1991;6;73-79.

von Frey M. Beitrage zur seenesphysiologice der haut. Ber d Kgl Sachs Ges D Eiss Math-Phys Kl 1895;47:166-184.

Weddell B. Somesthesis and the chemical senses. Annu Rev Psychol 1955;6:119-136.

Wells PE, Frampton V, Bowsher D. Pain management in physical therapy. Norwalk, CT: Appleton & Lange, 1988.

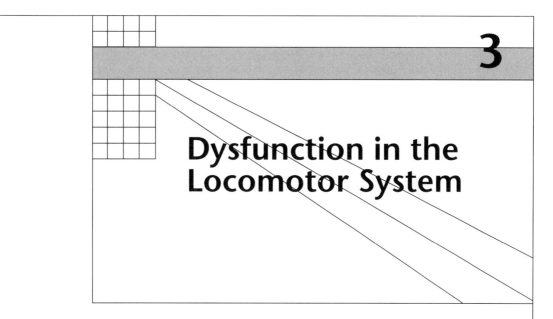

Dysfunction in the Locomotor System

Learning Objectives

At the completion of this chapter, you should be able to:

1. Describe the problems and alterations related to
   - joint dysfunction
   - muscular changes
   - myofascial changes
   - neuromuscular changes
2. Describe the various forms of treatment that are used to treat dysfunction.
3. Define a myofascial trigger point, listing its characteristics.
4. Describe the various grades of soft tissue injury.
5. Describe the various types of soft tissue injury.
6. Describe the severity ratings of soft tissue injury.

The neuromusculoskeletal system, otherwise known as the locomotor system, has been referred to as **"the primary machinery of life"** (Korr, 1978). It is through this system that life itself is expressed. It is undoubtedly more than coincidence that many of the descriptions of life and health that we use refer to this system. For example: "He has a spring in his step" may depict the individual who feels healthy, whereas: "He's all tied in knots" may be used to describe the individual who is stressed and tense. The chiropractor's approach to health care is unique in its emphasis on the health and function of the locomotor system. Perhaps more than anything else, this may represent the most significant difference between the chiropractor and the allopath.

Residual Changes

It is postulated that any change in the functional capabilities of the locomotor system will have an impact, not only on the muscles and joints, but on the quality of health of the individual. After the body has had a chance to respond to the initial phases of an injury, it passes through a period of recovery—the remodeling phase. During this phase the body attempts to restore both structure and function to as near normal as possible (SAID). Provided that the injury is not too severe, the individual is in relatively good health, and the care rendered is appropriate, remodeling is usually adequate for most circumstances. It is not unusual, however, to find residual dysfunction many years after an injury has occurred. This dysfunction may or may not be accompanied by pain. Often, when an event produces an exacerbation of this underlying problem, the patient seeks help from a chiropractor.

The residual changes that develop in the locomotor system may be relatively simple and easily remedied. In other instances, these changes may be extremely complicated and may affect multiple areas of the body. The problems may be categorized in the following areas: (1) joint dysfunction, (2) muscular changes, (3) myofascial changes, and (4) neuromuscular changes.

Joint Dysfunction

When a synovial joint is injured, such as in the patient who suffers a sprained ankle, the treatment typically follows a course of early immobilization and the application of ice. In fact, the classic form of treatment is described by the acronym RICE: rest, ice, compression, and elevation. As mentioned, the acute stage of injury lasts for approximately 2 to 3 days, after which there is a gradual lessening of symptoms and a return to activity. Treatment is often reduced or eliminated once the affected joint is free of pain. This may occur as soon as 1 week to 10 days. Treatment usually is directed at symptoms, often with little or no regard for any underlying functional problems.

Following a joint injury, it is not uncommon for an individual to complain of recurrent problems and weakening of the joint. For example, many patients express concern over the ease with which their ankle may be reinjured, and some modify their activities to reduce the likelihood of future problems. Even though the once-injured joint is no longer painful, evaluation of range of motion, strength, and balance indicates that recovery is not complete.

The changes that ensue in a synovial joint following injury usually involve a reduction of full range of motion (Figure 3.1), which may

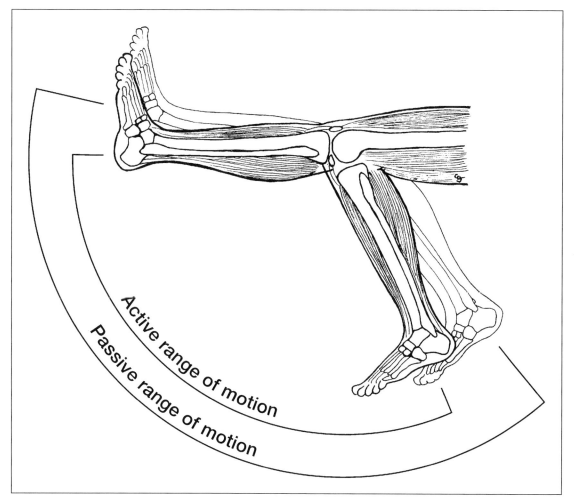

FIGURE 3.1   Normal range of motion of a synovial joint involves both active and passive components.

include **active range of motion, passive range of motion, joint play**, or a combination of all three. These changes are often due to a build-up of fibrous tissue and adhesions in the joint structures, and the patient may or may not be aware of the residual loss. Such range of motion loss may also be due to a change in joint kinematics or alignment. Obviously, any joint that is left in a state of reduced mobility (*i.e.*, **hypomobile**) will benefit from some increase in its range. Many studies have shown that early, gentle mobility exercises and procedures actually reduce the likelihood of residual changes as well as enhance the healing process (Salter, 1983).

Under some circumstances the range of motion of a joint may actually increase and the joint may be considered to be **hypermobile**. A **hypermobile joint** is one that exhibits more than its normal range of motion. Occasionally a joint may be left **unstable**. The term *unstable* refers to a joint that "**is no longer able to withstand normal physiologic stresses.**" This term often is used inappropriately and a clear distinction should be made between **instability** and **hypermobility**. An unstable joint can always be considered hypermobile, but not all hypermobile joints are unstable.

Joints that are left unstable as a result of injury or disease will benefit from therapeutic efforts to provide additional support. This support can come either in the form of increased muscle strength in the surrounding musculature (*e.g.*, strengthening exercises for the rotator cuff muscles following a shoulder dislocation) or from the addition of an external supporting device (*e.g.*, a Lennox-Hill brace for an unstable knee). Under some circumstances, surgery may be necessary to provide stability to unstable joints.

Treatment for the various articular changes involves:

- mobilization
- manipulation
- stretching and mobility exercises
- ultrasound
- shortwave diathermy
- paraffin baths
- electrical stimulation

Many of these (*e.g.*, ultrasound) are used in an attempt to make the tissues more pliable to manual procedures such as mobilization and manipulation or to reduce the pain and stiffness and make other treatment methods more comfortable. It should be emphasized that the use of such passive modalities plays a supportive rather than a primary therapeutic role.

Muscular Changes

As with the joint, the muscles in an injured area go through a similar remodeling phase. If the muscle is injured directly it too may become fibrotic. The developing scars may limit the muscle's ability to contract or to relax, resulting in a shortened, weakened muscle.

Even when a muscle is not directly injured, it may be adversely affected by the treatment, particularly by long periods of immobilization. Consider the patient who falls and breaks a wrist. The initial treatment involves immobilizing the broken bones for a period of 6 to 8 weeks. During this time the arm is supported by a sling and movement is minimal or absent in the entire upper limb. Following removal of the cast, the patient is left with joints in the wrist, hand, elbow, and shoulder that are less mobile than normal. Likewise, the muscles in the upper limb grow weak and short. Any attempt to rehabilitate the patient's wrist must include stretching and strengthening exercises for all of the joints and muscles throughout the entire affected limb (see Case 2, Chapter 1).

As a result of injury and of subsequent immobilization following injury, the muscles may become short, tight, weak, and imbalanced. Each specific type of change requires a particular type of treatment and exercise program to rehabilitate properly. Treatment methods directed at the muscular component include:

- active and passive stretching techniques
- muscle energy procedures
- stretching exercises
- strengthening exercises: isometric, isotonic, and isokinetic
- ultrasound
- moist heat
- shortwave diathermy
- electrical stimulation
- ice massage

Myofascial Changes

Important changes take place both in the muscle tissue itself and in the fascial tissues that surround the muscle. As with other injured tissues, these changes involve the invasion of fibrous tissue and adhesions. A common problem of muscular tissue is the development of **myofascial trigger points**. A trigger point is defined as "a local area of hyperirritability that, when provoked, refers pain, paraesthesia and autonomic symptoms to a location that is specific for the muscle" (Travell, Simons, 1983). Trigger points result in short, tight muscles; decreased range of motion; muscle weakness; and pain (Figure 3.2).

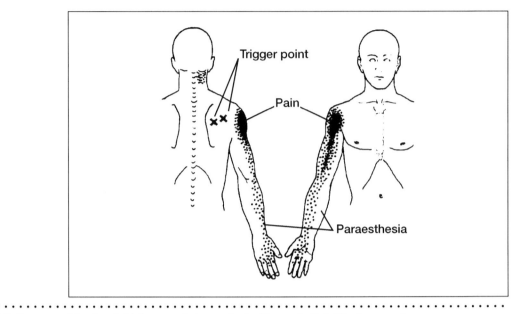

FIGURE 3.2   Myofascial trigger points are foci of hyperirritability in muscles.

Myofascial trigger points (TPs) are characterized by:

- characteristic patterns of pain that are specific to individual muscles
- weakness and restriction in the stretch range of motion of the affected muscle
- a taut, palpable band in the affected muscle
- exquisite, focal tenderness to digital pressure
- a local twitch response elicited through irritation of the tender spot
- reproduction of the patient's pain complaint by pressure on, or irritation of, the tender spot
- elimination of symptoms by therapy directed specifically at the affected muscle

For information regarding the location of myofascial trigger points, refer to Appendix B. Myofascial Trigger Point Locations.

Various treatment methods may be used to focus specifically on the trigger point; including:

- spray and stretch
- ultrasound stimulation
- electrical stimulation

- massage or digital pressure
- ice massage
- stretching exercises

The choice of treatment is often based on the location of the trigger point, the sensitivity of the patient, and the expertise and training of the clinician. For example, trigger points found in the upper trapezius and the levator scapulae may respond readily to digital pressure or to a combination of ultrasound and electrical stimulation. For obvious reasons, trigger points that are located in the anterior scalenes or the sternomastoid muscle should not be treated with such procedures. These muscles may be more appropriately treated with manual stretching techniques. It should be pointed out that whatever treatment mechanism is employed, ultimately the muscle containing the trigger points must be stretched (Figure 3.3). Other procedures employed are secondary to the stretching.

As with many other conditions, it is important for the chiropractor to address the underlying problems that led to the development of myofascial trigger points. Because many of the conditions associated with the devel-

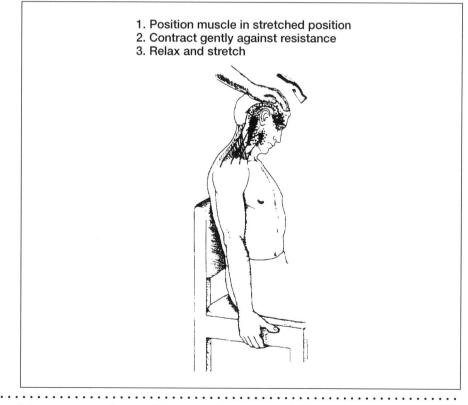

1. Position muscle in stretched position
2. Contract gently against resistance
3. Relax and stretch

FIGURE 3.3   Numerous muscle stretching procedures are available to the chiropractor.

opment of trigger points may have their origin in sustained postural stress of the affected muscle, it may be beneficial to evaluate the daily activities of the patient. Unless stressful postures are identified and modified, many patients may receive only temporary relief from their complaints. Consider the female patient who is suffering with problems resulting from trigger points in the upper back and shoulders. Her job requires her to spend several hours at a time working in a flexed, forward bent position at a work surface that is too high for her. Consequently, the upper trapezius, levator scapulae, deltoid, and supraspinatus muscles are constantly working. By the end of the work day she is sore and often complains of a headache. She has been treated in the past with a variety of procedures including moist heat, ultrasound, and therapeutic massage. Each time she expresses some immediate relief from her pain with treatment but is frustrated that her problems return in a day or two. It should be apparent that unless something is done to remove the causative factors (*i.e.*, sustained postural stress), the problem cannot be resolved. Treatment in such instances is purely symptomatic.

Neuromuscular Changes

The neural tissues and the neuromuscular coordination are often affected by both injury and treatment (*e.g.* immobilization) that ensues. Changes seen include a loss of neuromuscular coordination, balance, and proprioception. Proprioception is an area currently receiving a great deal of attention in the rehabilitation of injured athletes, and many conditions are being treated with some form of specific neuromuscular therapy. As an example, the downhill skier or the ballet dancer who fractures a leg must work to recover strength, range of motion, and balance. Exercises that are used to develop strength are different from those used to recover range of motion. In a similar context, exercises used to develop balance and coordination are different from those used to increase strength or improve range of motion.

Although it is commonplace to address issues of balance and coordination in the skier or dancer, similar efforts are not as common with an injury to a construction worker. If full recovery is desired, however, the same attention devoted to professional athletes should also be given to the "industrial athlete" or the "weekend warrior."

Some of the techniques used to rehabilitate the neuromuscular tissues include (Figure 3.4):

- proprioceptive neuromuscular facilitation (PNF)
- wobble board or balance board
- electrical stimulation

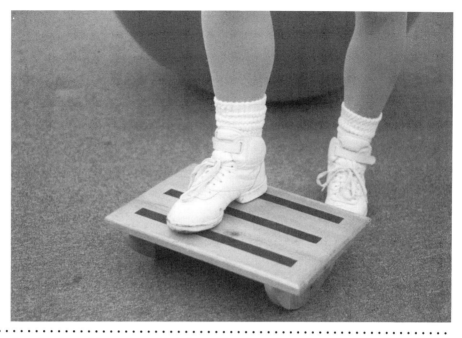

FIGURE 3.4 A rocker board is used to rehabilitate the neuromuscular tissues.

Soft Tissue Injuries

In the past, many clinicians have viewed the **soft tissue injury** with suspicion and disregard. Because many of these musculoskeletal injuries were difficult to detect on x-rays or to confirm with other tests, it was often assumed that they really did not exist. In other instances, injuries to the muscles or ligaments were simply viewed as unimportant. It is not uncommon for a patient to be evaluated with a variety of tests, including radiographs, after an injury. When no fracture, dislocation or pathology is seen, the patient often is told that there is "nothing really wrong." In other instances, the patient is told that the problem is "only a muscle" and, therefore, not really significant.

I recall seeing a young dancer who had recently injured her ankle rather seriously. She had been taken to a local emergency room for x-rays. Seeing no osseous changes, the attending physician told her that, "it wasn't really serious, only a ligament..." It is curious that a soft tissue injury such as a muscle spasm or ligament sprain in a professional athlete takes on a far more serious implication in the eye of the medical staff. A place kicker on a professional football team who develops a hamstring pull is treated with much greater concern than a warehouseman with a pulled muscle in his back. In the football player the injury will be viewed as a serious, potentially career-ending injury. Therapy will be aggressive and will include passive modalities and a graded exercise and stretching program. Only when the medical staff is confident that the player has recovered completely, will he be allowed to return to work. In the warehouseman, however, the worker may actually be largely ignored by the medical staff. In some instances, the existence of the injury may even be questioned. Therapy often includes muscle relaxants and rest, quite a different therapy plan than that seen for the athlete.

In spite of the past record of ignoring muscle and ligament problems, during the last several years greater attention has been placed on the nature of soft tissue injuries. It is now well recognized that, whereas these injuries may not show up on x-rays, they often cause serious pain and disability and may continue to create problems for years after an injury. As an example, many patients may continue to suffer from recurrent ankle injuries or back problems in spite of the fact that no fractures have been detected. In addition, with the development and increasing use of diagnostic tests such as the magnetic resonance imaging (MRI), our ability to visualize soft tissues has improved. As we learn to better assess such injuries, we have developed a better appreciation for them.

Grades of Soft Tissue Injuries

Soft tissue injuries include both those that affect muscles (**strains**) and those that affect ligaments (**sprains**). To develop appropriate treatment protocols, it is necessary to quantify the extent of damage that has been done. It is customary to classify the degree of strain or sprain injury to muscle and ligament as grade I, II, or III (Curl, 1990) and the nature of the injury as complicated or uncomplicated.

Grade I

This is described as a condition wherein the fibers of the muscle or ligament remain grossly intact, both anatomically and functionally. Most of these injuries resolve quickly without treatment.

General Qualities
Patients may complain of mild tenderness with some swelling.

Specific Qualities
Muscle. Passive stretch of the injured muscle is painless, whereas any resisted stretch is accompanied by pain. Full contracture of the muscle belly is evident and muscle strength is limited only by pain.

Ligament. Passive stretch is painful; however, very little or no instability of the joint is detected.

Grade II

This is a more serious condition wherein the fibers of the muscle or ligament are partially ruptured or torn. For the most part, the structure remains functionally intact. This classification probably represents most injuries to soft tissues and damage may vary from a small portion of the muscle or ligament (perhaps 10%) to a much larger portion (80% or more). Consequently, when an injury is described as a grade II sprain or strain, some additional term probably should be used to further qualify the extent of the injury (*e.g.*, moderate grade II sprain of the anterior cruciate ligament).

General Qualities

There is obvious swelling, ecchymosis, and functional difficulty. Patients often complain of pain with movement and activity. The more serious the injury, the greater the number of symptoms.

Specific Qualities

Muscle. Passive stretch of the muscle is painless versus painful resisted stretch. The pain that is elicited with resisted stretch is more severe than grade I and may vary greatly depending on the amount of muscle tearing. Partial areas of contracture of the muscle belly may be evident. Point tenderness to palpation demonstrates the site of the injury.

Ligament. Passive stretch is painful; however, mild to moderate instability of the joint may be evident. End-feel remains ligamentous in quality. X-ray stress tests may confirm the lesion.

Grade III

This is an advanced condition wherein the fibers of the muscle or ligament are completely ruptured or torn and the structure fails in a functional sense.

General Qualities

Swelling, hemorrhage, functional loss or gross instability is present. Not all grade III injuries are accompanied by pain.

Specific Qualities

Muscle. Passive stretch of the torn muscle is painless but the patient is unable to perform any resisted stretch. There is usually a deformity and a palpable defect will be noted.

Ligament. Passive stretch may not be painful depending on the area and surrounding damage. Gross instability of the joint is detected by orthopedic examination. Radiographic stress tests demonstrate the lesion.

Types of Soft Tissue Injuries

In addition to grading severity of injury, it is helpful to provide further clarification regarding the full extent of the injury and the presence of any complicating factors. The following is suggested.

Uncomplicated Injury

This is a confined or singular injury or injury complex that closely matches the mechanism of injury. For example, a patient who presents with a grade I ankle sprain may state that the ankle was twisted during a softball game. Although the injury was painful, it did not prevent the patient from continuing to participate in the game.

Complicated Injury

This represents a more extensive or complex injury that may involve a variety of body tissues. Some affected tissues may not correlate directly to the mechanism of injury or the problem may involve different tissue types (*e.g.*, bone) or different types of illness (*e.g.*, emotional overlay). An example is a grade II sprain of the lower back with a vertebral body compression fracture.

Severity Ratings of Soft Tissue Injuries

In addition to the above grading system, a subjective rating scale may also be applied to further describe the **severity** of injury and the degree of pain. The most commonly used terms are minimal, mild, moderate, and severe.

Minimal Injury
Such an injury does not usually require treatment. The person is able to continue with all activities of daily living (ADL) and the condition resolves quickly.

Minimal Pain
This does not cause suffering and does not interfere with the person's emotional status. The injured individual usually does not seek professional help.

Mild Injury
Mild injury may or may not require treatment. The person is able to continue with most, if not all, ADL. Treatment is brief and usually successful.

Mild Pain
Mild pain does cause some suffering and may, rarely, interfere with the person's emotional status. Any changes usually are temporary.

Moderate Injury

This type of injury typically requires treatment. Some ADL are affected. The treatment usually takes weeks to a few months; it should include periodic re-evaluation and has clear treatment objectives. Treatment methods change as the patient progresses through the various stages of recovery.

Moderate Pain

Moderate pain causes suffering and may interfere with emotional status. It usually prompts a person to seek treatment.

Severe Injury

This is a life-threatening, potentially mutilating, disfiguring, or otherwise serious injury. Such a designation should be reserved for "emergency" or urgent care situations. These conditions are not likely to be seen by the chiropractor. It may be acceptable to add the term **form** of a mild or moderate injury (*e.g.*, a severe form of a moderate cervical myofascial pain syndrome).

Severe Pain

Severe pain that causes intense suffering and by itself functionally disables the patient. The pain is excruciating and the patient is in acute distress. Although severe injuries are not often seen in the chiropractic office, some chiropractic patients may have severe pain. The patient who is disabled with an acute intervertebral disc herniation may have severe pain for a few days. Fortunately, such patients typically improve quickly in the chiropractor's office.

Summary

This section described the body's initial reaction to injury, the healing process, the problem of pain, and the resulting problems that develop in the musculoskeletal tissues as a result of both the injury and the treatment process itself. Treatment must be directed at the specific changes that have developed and may develop and should be based on some understanding of the conditions at hand and on the physiologic effects of the treatment methods employed. As the condition changes, so must the treatment.

References and Suggested Reading

Curl DD. Soft tissue injuries (Seminar Notes). Los Angeles: Los Angeles College of Chiropractic, 1990.

Korr IM (ed.). Neurobiologic mechanisms in manipulative therapy. New York: Plenum Press, 1978.

Salter R. Textbook of disorders of the musculoskeletal system. Baltimore: Williams and Wilkins, 1983.

Travell JG, Simons DG. Myofascial pain and dysfunction: the trigger point manual. Baltimore: Williams and Wilkins, 1983.

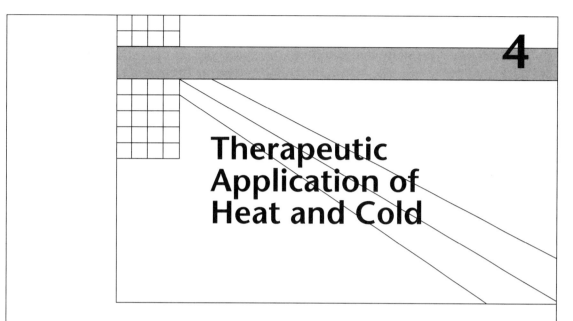

Therapeutic Application of Heat and Cold

4

Learning Objectives

At the completion of this chapter, you should be able to:

1. Describe the electromagnetic spectrum.
2. Describe the various methods by which radiant energy is conducted, providing examples of each.
3. Describe what happens to radiant energy when it strikes tissue.
4. Describe the laws of physics as they affect radiant energy.
5. Define the following:
   - cosine law
   - inverse square rule
   - Law of Grotthus Draper
   - Arndt-Schultz principle
6. Describe the following thermal modalities that are commonly used in physical therapy. Include a discussion of the physiologic effects, indications and contraindications, application techniques, and precautions:
   - cryotherapy
   - paraffin baths
   - hydrocollator packs
   - whirlpools

- infrared lamps
- ultraviolet light
7. List five contraindications for the use of each of the various forms of heat and cold; describe the reason for any contraindication.
8. Describe the general guidelines for using heat and cold in patient care with particular attention to the variations in use that accompany the different stages of injury.
9. Differentiate between the following:
   - general contraindication to treatment
   - absolute contraindication to treatment
   - treatment that is not indicated
10. Describe the various stages of burn injuries.

A variety of applications of heat and cold have been used in attempts to alleviate pain and suffering through time. Ancient dissertations on medical problems show that ice and cold water were used to treat fevers and headaches, whereas heat was used to treat arthritis, lumbago, and rheumatism. Many of these applications are still popular, especially for home care. More recently, some rather sophisticated devices have been developed to administer thermal energy in an effort to relieve aches and pains. Even so, with all the advances of modern science, there is probably no single therapy that is more common than the tried and true hot-water bottle.

In a general sense, the use of thermal agents in physical therapy can be placed in two broad categories: (1) those capable of exerting an effect only on the more superficial tissues and (2) those capable of exerting a direct effect on the deeper tissues (*i.e.*, the diathermies). In this chapter we will discuss those modalities in the first category, the superficial thermal agents. Each of these modalities represents a type of electromagnetic energy and falls in the **infrared** portion of the electromagnetic spectrum. To better understand the effects of the various forms of superficial heat and cold, it is first necessary to review the physical properties of electromagnetic energy.

Electromagnetic Spectrum

When a sufficient chemical or electrical force is applied to an object, the resulting movement of electrons creates the various forms of electromagnetic energy. **Electromagnetic energy** is defined by the range of frequencies and wavelengths associated with radiant energy and includes each of the following: electrical stimulating currents, shortwave and microwave diathermy, the infrared modalities, ultraviolet light, and x-rays (Figure 4.1).

Portion of the Electromagnetic Spectrum	Wavelength	Frequency	Physiologic Effect
Electrical stimulating currents	3×10^8 Km to 75,000 Km	1 to 4000 Hz	Pain reduction, muscle contraction, edema reduction
Commercial radio and television			
Shortwave diathermy	22 m 11 m	13.56 MHz 27.12 MHz	Increased temperature of deep tissues, vasodilation, increased blood flow
Microwave diathermy	33 cm 12 cm	915 MHz 2450 MHz	Increased temperature of deep tissues, vasodilation, increased blood flow
Infrared portion Cold packs Cold whirlpool	111,000 A 99,500 A	2.7×10^{12} Hz 3.0×10^{12} Hz	Superficial temperature reduction, vasoconstriction, decreased blood flow, analgesia
Hot whirlpool Paraffin bath Hydrocollator Luminous IR lamp Non-luminous IR	93,000 A 90,200 A 82,500 A 28,800 A 14,400 A	3.2×10^{12} Hz 3.3×10^{12} Hz 3.6×10^{12} Hz 1.0×10^{12} Hz 2.1×10^{12} Hz	Superficial temperature elevation, vasodilation, increased blood flow
Ultraviolet	3200-2900 A	9.38×10^{13} - 1.03×10^{14} Hz	Superficial chemical changes, tanning, bactericidal effects
Ionizing radiation (x-rays, gamma rays)			

FIGURE 4.1   The electromagnetic spectrum is comprised of various forms of radiant energy.

Each of the various types of radiant energy is classified according to its position on the electromagnetic spectrum. This position is determined by analyzing the wavelength and frequency of the energy.

Wavelength is defined as the distance between the peak of one wave and the peak of a subsequent wave. **Frequency** is defined as the number of waves or oscillations occurring in 1 second. Frequency is expressed in **hertz (Hz)**. There is an inverse relationship between wavelength and frequency (Figure 4.2). This relationship may be expressed as:

Velocity = wavelength × frequency

Regardless of the form of radiant energy, all types of electromagnetic radiation travel at a similar velocity (approximately 300,000 meters/second). Therefore, those energy forms with short wavelengths have long frequencies and those with longer wavelengths have shorter frequencies.

Radiation is a process by which electromagnetic energy travels through space. All forms of radiant energy travel in a straight line. However, when the energy strikes an object such as the human body it may be modified in a number of ways. It may be bent or refracted as when a beam of light passes through a prism. It may be reflected as when light strikes a mirror. The energy may penetrate the target similar to light passing through clear glass or it may be absorbed (Figure 4.3). The particular reaction is dependent on several factors, including the wavelength and frequency of the energy and the particular structure of the objects in the path of the energy.

Radiant energy can be transmitted through space by several means:

1. It can be **conducted** through the contact of two objects at different temperatures. An example of conduction is seen in the application

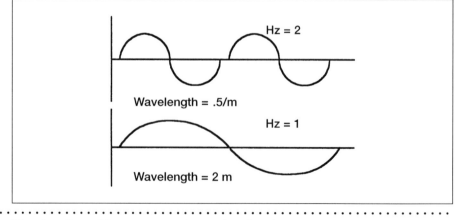

FIGURE 4.2   Wavelength and frequency are inversely related.

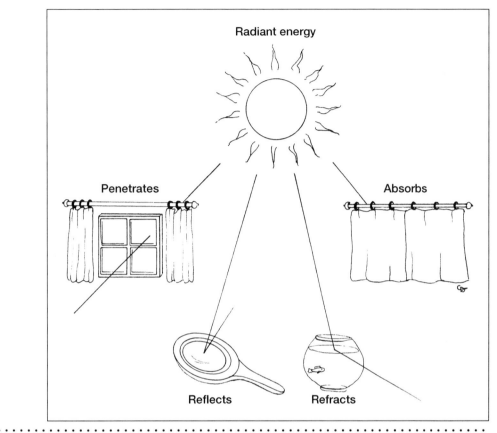

Radiant energy

Penetrates

Absorbs

Reflects

Refracts

FIGURE 4.3   Object struck by radiant energy may be modified in a number of ways.

of a hydrocollator pack or ice pack that is placed directly in contact with the patient. The hydrocollator conducts thermal energy to the patient whereas the ice pack conducts energy away from the patient.

2. Energy can be transmitted through the movement of heated air or water. This is referred to as **convection**. An example of convection is seen in a whirlpool or in fluidotherapy (heated air). We are probably most familiar with convection currents as they apply to air and water, which are frequently used to explain changes in weather patterns.

3. Finally, electromagnetic energy can be altered or changed into mechanical energy, which in turn produces thermal energy in the form of heat. This process is referred to as **conversion**. An example

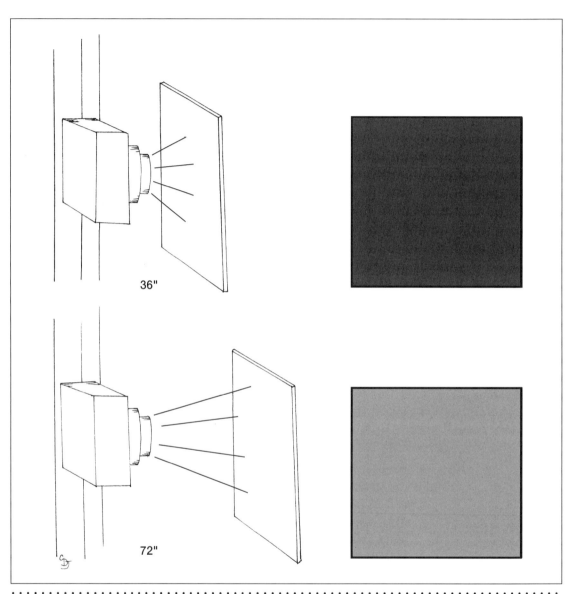

FIGURE 4.4   Inverse square law: the intensity of radiant energy is inversely proportional to the square of the distance from the source to the target.

of energy conversion is seen in the shortwave and microwave diathermies. The high frequency electromagnetic energy produced by these devices causes molecular vibration in tissues. The resulting friction caused by these vibrating molecules produces heat in the deeper tissues of the body.

Inverse Square Law

All forms of radiant energy are subject to **the inverse square law**. This law states that the intensity of radiation is inversely proportional to the square of the distance from the source of energy to the target. In other words, the closer the source of energy to the target, the greater the energy. An example of the inverse square law is seen in the tube-to-film distance used in taking radiographs (Figure 4.4). Doubling the tube-to-film distance from 36 to 72 inches reduces the power of the x-ray beam by one fourth.

Cosine Law

Radiant energy is also subject to **the cosine law** that states that energy at right angles to the target has the greatest effect. Conversely, the greater the angle at which the energy strikes the target, the less the intensity. An infrared lamp placed parallel to the skin exerts much less effect than one placed at a 90 degree angle. Likewise, x-rays at other than a 90 degree angle from the target are much more likely to be deflected or absorbed. The cosine law can be demonstrated with the x-ray beam. Those rays that strike the body at angles other than 90 degrees are absorbed or deflected much more readily (Figure 4.5).

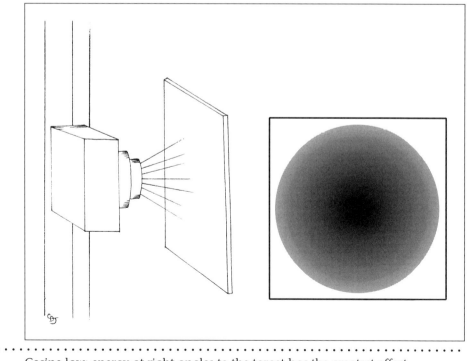

FIGURE 4.5   Cosine law: energy at right angles to the target has the greatest effect.

Law of Grotthus-Draper

Any energy that is not absorbed by the superficial tissues is transmitted to the deeper layers of tissue. For obvious reasons, the greater the amount of energy that is absorbed, the less is transmitted and penetrates. One of the primary clinical problems with most of the infrared modalities is the loss of energy in the superficial tissues. For all practical purposes, no infrared modality is capable of eliciting a direct effect on tissues at a depth exceeding 10 mm. Consequently, when it is necessary to increase the temperatures of the deeper tissues, other forms of therapy must be used (*e.g.*, diathermy or ultrasound) (Figure 4.6).

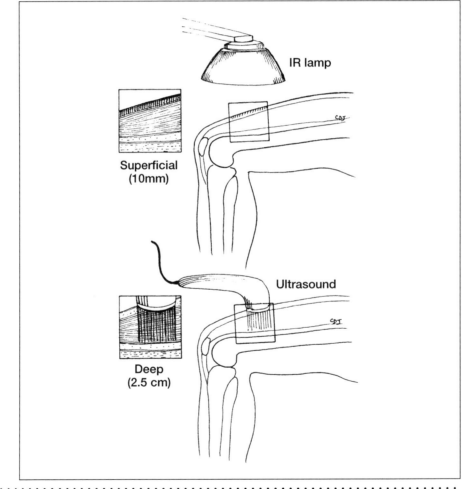

FIGURE 4.6   Law of Grotthus-Draper: radiant energy from superficial thermal agents is absorbed before it reaches the deeper tissues.

Arndt-Schultz Principle

Because the primary goal in using radiant energy is to produce a reaction in the tissues being treated, it is imperative that the energy be sufficient to stimulate the desired reaction. The **Arndt-Schultz principle** states that no reactions will occur unless there is sufficient energy to stimulate the absorbing tissues. A good example of this may be seen in the use of a subthreshold electrical current. Such a current does not produce any effect on neurologic tissues and cannot produce a sensory response or muscle contraction (Figure 4.7).

Infrared Modalities

The infrared portion of the electromagnetic spectrum consists of that portion with wavelengths and frequencies found between the diathermies and ultraviolet light (see Fig. 4.1). The therapeutic modalities in the infrared portion of the spectrum are used to produce both local and generalized heating or cooling of the superficial body tissues. These modalities are all considered superficial thermal agents because the energy produced is only capable of penetrating the body to a depth of approximately 1 cm. Within this range, the wavelengths are temperature-dependent, with those modalities at the lowest temperatures having the longest wavelength. Because longer wavelengths are associated with a greater depth of penetration, ice packs have a greater direct effect on the deeper tissues than hydrocollator packs. High temperature modalities such as infrared lamps have an extremely superficial effect.

In general, each of the infrared modalities can elicit either an increase or a decrease in circulation, both locally and generally. In addition, they also have some analgesic effects and alter the viscosity of blood and body fluids. They may also exert a general relaxing effect on the patient. Because relaxation of tight muscles is often one of the primary reasons for using superficial heat, it should be pointed out that any relaxation achieved is not the result of any significant increase in the temperature of muscle. Rather, relaxation of tight muscles is due to a general relaxation of the body when exposed to warm temperatures. The limited ability of these modalities to alter the temperature of the deeper tissues must be emphasized.

Superficial Thermal Agents

Superficial thermal agents are found in the infrared portion of the electromagnetic spectrum. They include those modalities that either increase or decrease the temperature of the superficial tissues of the body. The thermal agents in this category include:

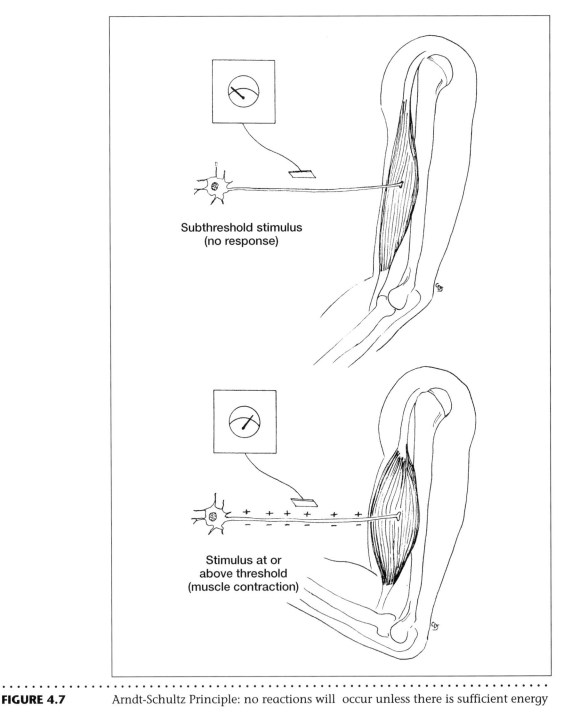

Subthreshold stimulus
(no response)

Stimulus at or
above threshold
(muscle contraction)

FIGURE 4.7   Arndt-Schultz Principle: no reactions will occur unless there is sufficient energy to stimulate the absorbing tissues.

- ice packs
- cold whirlpools
- warm whirlpools
- paraffin baths
- hydrocollator packs
- infrared heat lamps

Cryotherapy

One of the most widely used therapies involves the application of various forms of cold, particularly ice. This is referred to as **cryotherapy** and includes the common ice pack, cold spray, cold whirlpools, and ice massage. It is almost universally agreed that the application of cold is indicated to treat most acute musculoskeletal injuries such as strains, sprains, and contusions. In fact, the traditional rule of treatment for an acute injury is **RICE**. This includes the application of **r**est, **i**ce, **c**ompression, and **e**levation. Anyone who has played some type of sport or who has watched someone play a sport, has seen an injured athlete on the sidelines with an ice pack on an injured limb. Ice is also used during the acute phase of many inflammatory conditions such as bursitis, tendinitis, and capsulitis.

The primary rationale for applying ice is the initial vasoconstriction that accompanies its use. The resulting reduction in blood flow assists in controlling swelling and edema that typifies the acute injury. In addition, ice also is used to reduce pain and muscle spasm. Cold, in the form of ice massage or vapocoolant spray, is also used as an adjunct in the treatment of many myofascial pain syndromes (*e.g.*, myofascial trigger points).

Reaction to Cold

The body responds to the application of ice in stages. The initial reaction to cold is local vasoconstriction with a consequent reduction in blood flow. This is useful during the early stage (*i.e.*, acute stage) when it is necessary to control swelling, which is the primary rationale for the use of ice immediately following an injury. In addition to reducing blood flow and fluid accumulation, ice also has an analgesic effect and is often used more to reduce pain than to minimize edema.

The initial period of vasoconstriction is followed rather quickly (within the first 15 to 30 minutes) by periods of intermittent vasodilation and vasoconstriction, each lasting from 4 to 6 minutes. This cyclic reaction is referred to as the "hunting" reaction and is a necessary response by the body to prevent tissue injury. With continued cooling the blood vessels in the affected tissues become maximally dilated.

Although there is a great variation in individual reactions to cryotherapy, the physiologic processes are consistent from one patient to another. With the application of cold the patient should experience the following stages: (1) a sensation of cold, (2) tingling or itching, (3) a burning or aching, and finally (4) numbness or anesthesia. Patients should be instructed about the sensations that they may expect as well as the relative time frame for each occurrence. As with other modalities or treatment methods, whenever ice is used for the first time, the patient should be monitored to ensure an appropriate response.

Physiologic Effects of Cooling

As stated, the response to cooling is consistent from one patient to another. The primary effects of the application of cold are:

- a local decrease in tissue temperature
- reduction in metabolism
- vasoconstriction (initially)
- reduced blood flow (initially)
- reduced nerve conduction velocity
- reduction in lymphatic and venous drainage
- reduced muscle excitability
- reduced muscle spindle activity
- decreased formation and accumulation of edema
- anesthesia

Clinical Application of Cold

Ice Packs
Application of ice packs is the most common form of cryotherapy. Although there is some disagreement regarding the correct application of ice packs, the following rules provide some useful guidelines:

1. Ice should be used during the acute stage (typically the first 48 to 72 hours) following an injury.
2. Fifteen to 20 minutes is adequate for most therapeutic applications; in fact, longer applications may actually create problems.
3. Applications should be repeated approximately every 2 hours as needed.
4. To reduce edema in a limb, ice should be used in conjunction with compression; in most instances, it is probably more productive to leave a properly applied compression device on for 24 hours or longer than to remove it to reapply ice.
5. Patient tolerance to ice varies considerably and must be taken into account.

Note: It is helpful to keep a supply of reusable ice packs of various sizes on hand. These packs may be provided to patients as a convenience. The patient may be sent home with two ice packs of equal size and should be instructed to place both ice packs in the freezer compartment of the refrigerator. Take out one of the ice packs when needed, wrap it in a dry towel and apply it to the appropriate body part. Return the ice pack to the freezer after 15 minutes. The second ice pack will be ready for use when it is time to reapply ice. It is also helpful to provide the patient with written instructions regarding the application of ice at home.

Note: It has been my experience that patient compliance with the use of ice as a form of home therapy is not particularly good. Because the use of ice is uncomfortable, patients often apply it for only short periods of time; in many instances, they do not use it at all.

Ice Massage

Ice massage is most popular in athletes, especially when stretching is a desired outcome. It can be performed by a therapist or as a self-treatment technique. Ice massage also is used as a substitute for the vapocoolant, fluoromethane (Figure 4.8) spray and stretch technique that was made popular by Travell and Simons.

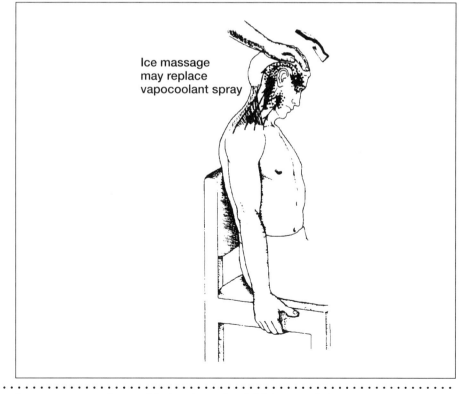

Ice massage
may replace
vapocoolant spray

FIGURE 4.8   Ice massage can be used to treat myofascial trigger points.

The following guidelines are suggested:

1. Use a styrofoam cup filled with water that has been placed in the freezer for several hours. Remove the bottom 1 inch of the cup and invert over the patient.
2. Apply the ice cup in a rotating pattern or in overlapping longitudinal strokes for approximately 10 to 15 minutes, or until the area is sufficiently anesthetized to allow adequate stretching.
3. Follow the application with stretching exercises, either active or passive.

Note: Applying ice directly to the skin with an ice massage results in significant reddening of the area treated. If any mottled or blanched areas appear, this treatment should be discontinued.

Cold Spray

The use of vapocoolant sprays such as fluoromethane was once very common. Today, based on concern both for the carcinogenic and environmental effects of fluorocarbons, their use is diminishing. However, these sprays are still used to treat myofascial trigger points and, when used sparingly, add a useful modality to the clinician's treatment armamentarium. Cold spray is indicated when stretching of an injured part is desired. These cold sprays do not provide the same type of physiologic response as the application of ice. Rather than exerting a thermal response that is similar to the application of other forms of cold, the cold spray serves as a counterirritant that distracts the patient's attention from sore muscles. This allows the patient to relax and facilitates the stretching process. The primary action of a cold spray is the breaking of the **pain-spasm-pain** cycle that often accompanies prolonged postural or physical stresses.

Note: Janet Travell made the use of vapocoolant spray commonplace for the treatment of myofascial trigger points. She often stated that "spray is distraction, stretch is action."

The following is a suggested procedure for the use of the vapocoolant spray on myofascial trigger points (Figure 4.9):

1. Spray the part with the fluoromethane spray in slow sweeping strokes.
2. The strokes should be directed from the trigger point toward the area of symptoms as shown.
3. Following the spray technique, the involved muscle should be passively stretched.
4. The procedure should be repeated two to three times at a setting.
5. Following the spray and stretch procedure, the involved muscle should be warmed with a hydrocollator pack or a heating pad.

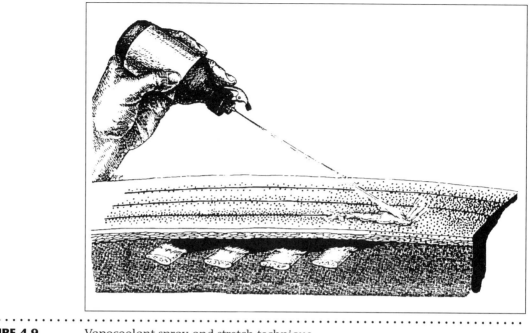

FIGURE 4.9   Vapocoolant spray and stretch technique.

Note: Because the fluoromethane that is used in the spray and stretch techniques is a fluorocarbon and a potential carcinogen, its use has diminished. It is more appropriate to use ice massage as described above as a substitute for the fluoromethane spray whenever possible. There are, however, instances where the spray is still a useful therapeutic tool. These include trigger points found in areas such as the sternomastoid and scalene muscles where the direct application of ice is not warranted.

Cold Whirlpool

The cold whirlpool is indicated in the treatment of an acute or subacute condition whenever exercise of the injured part during cold application is desired. The following should be considered:

1. A temperature of 50°F to 60°F should be used.
2. The water temperature should be between 65°F to 80°F for total body immersion.
3. Treatment time should not exceed 15 minutes.

Contrast Therapy

In most instances, cold is recommended as a treatment for the inflammation and swelling that accompany an acute injury. During the later stages of healing and repair, when it is helpful to warm tissues prior to stretching, mobilization, manipulation or exercise, heat is often applied. Between these two phases, however, there is a transitional period during which it may be helpful to apply both ice and heat. Alternating applications of ice and heat is referred to as **contrast therapy** and is directed at improving the circulation in injured tissues.

The application of contrast therapy involves several different methods, but probably is most appropriately performed in the following manner:

1. Two containers are used. One is filled with cold water (50°F to 60°F), the second with warm water (104°F to 106°F).
2. Immerse the injured area in the cold water for a period of 1 minute.
3. Remove the injured area from the cold water bath and immerse it in the warm water for a period of 3 minutes.
4. Reimmerse the part in the cold water bath and repeat the procedure five times.

Note: It is important to maintain the temperature of the water during the treatment time.

A second, more practical method of contrast therapy that can be used by a patient at home involves alternating applications of ice packs and heat packs. The patient should be instructed to apply ice for 5 minutes, followed by heat for 5 minutes. This should be repeated two times for a total treatment time of 20 minutes. It is necessary that the patient have two ice packs and two heat packs for this procedure.

Although contrast therapy is clinically effective, there are some significant disadvantages that make it a relatively uncommon form of therapy. Most importantly, the procedure is messy and somewhat cumbersome. Consequently, it is not a widespread form of therapy.

Indications

A number of conditions may be effectively treated by applying various forms of cold. The following conditions and symptoms are considered reasonable indications for the application of ice:

- to reduce bleeding after injury
- to reduce swelling and edema
- to reduce muscle spasms
- to reduce blood flow to inflamed areas
- burns
- to reduce blood flow and metabolism in insect or snake bites
- boils and carbuncles
- fevers
- herpes blisters

Contraindications

Certain problems may not be helped by the application of ice and the various forms of cold therapy. Others may actually be worsened through such procedures. The following conditions and symptoms are considered contraindications for the use of cryotherapy:

- Raynaud's disease
- rheumatoid or gouty arthritis
- frostbite or chilblains
- sensory deficits
- paroxysmal cold hemoglobinuria

Superficial Heat

As with the widespread use of ice packs, one of the most common and most popular forms of therapy is the application of various forms of heat. Ranging from the warm poultice to the hot water bottle or the electric blanket, this comfortable form of therapy has been used by individuals for many years. Although clinically heat applications do not typically have any profound physiologic effect, one of the reasons for its widespread application is the high degree of patient comfort that is associated with gentle heat. Unlike the application of ice, heat is usually well received by patients.

Reaction to Heat

The local application of heat is recommended in many subacute or chronic conditions to reduce pain and inflammation and to increase blood flow and venous return. Superficial heating produces a change both in the local tissue and in tissues at a distance to the injury. Heat causes vasodilation and a subsequent increase in local blood flow; it also increases the elasticity of connective tissue and facilitates stretching of shortened tissues. In addition, there is an increase in the metabolic rate of heated tissue that is proportional to the increase in temperature.

Both heat and cold appear to have an effect on the receptors within a muscle. Heat is said to lessen the threshold of the muscle spindles and to decrease the firing rate of the gamma efferent fibers, resulting in a relaxed state.

Note: I have felt for a long time that the relaxation that accompanies the application of moist heat packs results from more than just a warming of the tissues. When patients present in a clinic for treatment they are often in a state of anxiety. Lying in a comfortable position on a therapy table with a moist heat pack in place has a direct effect on the superficial tissues. This may be accompanied by a change in nerve activity within the muscles that results from warming. In addition, however, the act of lying in a comfortable position for 20 minutes also has a relaxing effect on many patients. It is suggested that the relaxation that accompanies such applications of moist heat is the result of a combined effect of warming and mental relaxation and not simply an increase in tissue temperature.

Physiologic Effects of Heating

As with cryotherapy, the body's response to warming is consistent from patient to patient. The primary effects of superficial heating are:

- local increase in tissue temperature
- increase in metabolism
- vasodilation
- increased blood flow
- increased capillary permeability
- increased lymphatic and venous drainage
- increased production of metabolites
- increased axon reflex activity
- increased elasticity of connective tissue
- increased formation of edema
- decreased muscle tone
- decrease in muscle spasm
- analgesia

Clinical Application of Superficial Heat

Moist Heat Packs

The application of moist heat is one of the most common of all physical therapies and has even been reported in ancient medical textbooks. Moist heat packs (hydrocollator packs) are used to relax patients, to increase local and peripheral circulation, and to reduce muscle spasm and tonicity. Commercially available heat packs (**hydrocollators**) consist of sand-filled bags that are kept in a water bath. The temperature of the water is maintained at a constant 170°F. Once removed from the water bath, the hot packs are wrapped in several layers of toweling (**6 layers or 1 inch**) and are applied for a period of 20 to 30 minutes (Figure 4.10). It is important that patients be monitored periodically to ensure that they are responding appropriately to the moist heat application. The normal response involves a gentle reddening (**erythema**) of the skin under the hot pack. If this reddening is mottled or uneven it may indicate an abnormal response to heating and therapy should be discontinued.

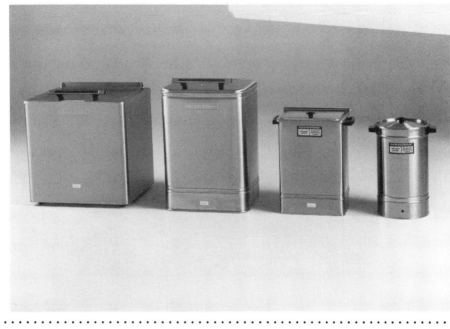

FIGURE 4.10   Hydrocollator pack consists of sand-filled bags that are kept in a water bath.

Note: Burns are one of the most common misuses of physical therapy that results in a significant number of injuries and subsequent malpractice suits. Inadequate protection of the patient's skin during the application of a moist heat pack (hydrocollator pack) is one way that this occurs. This may be particularly problematic in elderly patients or in patients who have any form of sensory deficit.

Note: It may be helpful to emphasize that moist heat packs are a form of superficial heat. The direct effect of these modalities is limited to the superficial tissues only.

Paraffin Baths

The paraffin bath is one of the most useful of the superficial thermal modalities. It is an easy, economical, and efficient way of applying gentle heat to an irregular surface such as the hand or wrist. The paraffin bath consists of a pan containing melted paraffin (candle wax) that is held at a constant temperature of approximately 126°F to 130°F (Figure 4.11). Perhaps the primary disadvantage of the paraffin bath is the limited number of areas that it can be used on.

The procedure for using a paraffin bath is as follows:

1. The part to be treated (*e.g.,* the hand) is immersed in the paraffin bath and then withdrawn.

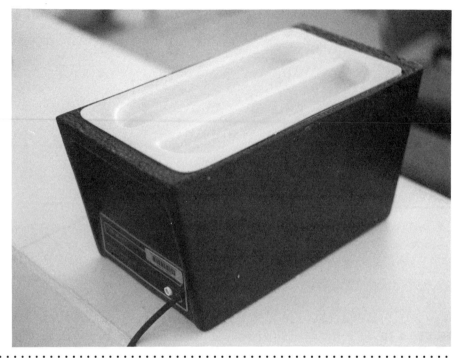

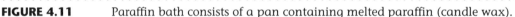

FIGURE 4.11   Paraffin bath consists of a pan containing melted paraffin (candle wax).

2. The warm coating of melted paraffin is allowed to cool for several seconds.

3. The hand is then reimmersed in the melted paraffin and withdrawn again.

4. This procedure is repeated 8 to 10 times.

5. The hand is then wrapped in cellophane and a dry towel and the heat is applied for approximately 20 to 30 minutes.

6. After the treatment the paraffin is removed and replaced in the bath.

7. Once the paraffin is removed the treated limb is exercised, stretched, or mobilized.

Note: This may be a particularly effective treatment aid for patients with arthritis of the hands and fingers and makes home exercise for stiff joints more comfortable and effective. The paraffin bath can be used in home care by instructing the patient to place candle wax in a crock-pot that is set at 125°F. Patients should be encouraged to use the warm paraffin several times a day to facilitate home stretching and exercise.

Warm Whirlpools

Whirlpools are often used in situations when heat needs to be combined with exercise. A common therapeutic use of warm water can be seen in the sitz bath used in the postpartum treatment of episiotomies. The whirlpool must be large enough to hold the body part to be treated and the following guidelines should be followed.

1. Temperature should be 98°F to 110°F for treatment of the arm and hand, 98°F to 104°F for treatment of the leg and foot, and 98°F to 102°F for full body treatment.
2. Treatment time should be between 15 and 20 minutes.
3. Patients should be placed in a comfortable position in the whirlpool.
4. The water in the whirlpool should be changed regularly to avoid bacterial contamination.

Infrared Lamps

The use of radiant heating lamps, both luminous (those that glow) and non-luminous (those that do not glow) is declining. These once popular modalities are now most often found in fast food restaurants and in many modern bathrooms and are used to keep food warm or to warm the air in a room. Although these lamps provide a gentle warming of the body, they have little therapeutic benefit owing to their extremely superficial effect on body tissues.

When used in a clinical setting, the lamps are placed at a distance of approximately 20 inches from the part to be heated and the body part is protected by a single layer of moist toweling (Figure 4.12). The heat is applied for 20 to 30 minutes. It is important to note that the surface of the lamp is extremely hot (approximately 4000°F) and direct patient contact with it should be avoided.

The primary advantage of such a heating device is that the patient is not touched by the lamp. Consequently, it is a hygienic method of heating superficial tissues. In addition, it may be useful for treatment of patients who cannot tolerate direct contact with a hydrocollator pack. The primary disadvantage of the infrared heating lamp is its extremely limited application. The depth of penetration is less than 1 mm and its effect is minimal.

Fluidotherapy

Fluidotherapy employs a stream of dry, heated air that passes over the injured body part. The injured body part can be exercised during the application of dry heat. It is very similar in concept to the exercises performed while in a warm whirlpool, but it is probably more hygienic. The temperature of the air is maintained between 110°F to 125°F and the treatment is applied for 15 to 20 minutes. This particular modality is uncommon in the chiropractic clinic.

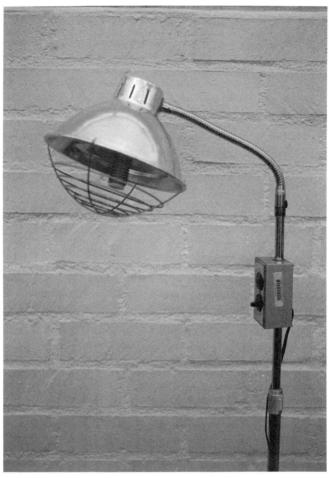

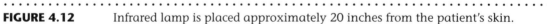

FIGURE 4.12   Infrared lamp is placed approximately 20 inches from the patient's skin.

Indications

The following conditions and symptoms are considered reasonable indications for the application of superficial heat:

- to increase hyperemia and blood flow
- to increase the threshold of pain receptors
- to increase local circulatory and metabolic rates
- to decrease vascular stasis
- to increase urinary output

- to enhance the absorption of exudates and metabolites
- to enhance local nutrition
- to increase lymphatic flow
- to increase pulse rate and cardiac volume
- to promote sweating
- to produce general sedation and local analgesia
- to increase the elasticity of connective tissues

Contraindications

The following conditions and symptoms are considered contraindications for the use of superficial heat:

- areas of diminished sensation
- malignancy
- patients receiving radiation therapy
- patients with bleeding tendencies
- patients with fevers
- patients with peripheral neuropathies
- patients with peripheral vascular diseases
- in infants, the elderly, or other patients who may be incapable of providing appropriate feedback
- over the pregnant uterus
- over acute inflammatory disorders (especially those involving suppurative lesions)
- over localized edema
- over skin rashes or open wounds
- over metal objects

Ultraviolet Light

Although the use of ultraviolet light was fairly common in the past, its application currently is limited to selected dermatologic conditions such as acne and psoriasis. It is not found in many chiropractic clinics, but will be discussed here for historical purposes. Although not a form of superficial heat or cold, the **ultraviolet** portion of the electromagnetic spectrum lies in close proximity to the infrared portion. The primary effects of ultraviolet light are photochemical and are seen in a reddening or tanning of the skin. Other effects are:

- increased formation of vitamin D
- increased formation of red blood cells
- bactericidal
- increase in cellular activity

Because of the danger of skin burns (sunburn), care should be exercised when patients are exposed to ultraviolet radiation. Exposure times must be closely monitored to reduce the possibility of problems. The following **sleeve test** is suggested to determine the exposure rate:

1. Cover the patient's skin with a cloth or a piece of cardboard that has five or six small openings.
2. Set the ultraviolet lamp 30 inches (hot quartz) or 1 inch (cold quartz) from the skin.
3. Expose each of the openings to varying applications of ultraviolet light (5-second intervals).
4. The **minimal erythemal dose (MED)** is that area that reddens after 8 hours and disappears after 24 hours.
5. Once the MED has been determined, it is safe to expose the patient to an additional 15 seconds with each successive treatment.

Stages of Erythema

Whenever cutaneous tissue is exposed to heat or to ultraviolet radiation, whether for therapeutic reasons or not, it reacts in a similar manner. The nature of the reaction is governed by several factors including both the duration and the intensity of the energy. If too much energy is supplied, injury occurs. If insufficient energy is supplied, the body fails to respond.

The following list provides a description of the superficial response to ultraviolet light and to other forms of heat.

First Degree. The minimal erythemal dose, this is seen as a slight reddening of the skin, without desquamation.

Second Degree. This is similar to a mild sunburn. There is a reddening of the skin that is followed by some desquamation and itching.

Third Degree. This involves a marked reddening with edema and blistering. There is a significant peeling and marked discomfort.

Fourth Degree. Intense reddening within several hours of exposure, followed by blistering and peeling. Marked tissue damage.

Indications

The following conditions and symptoms are considered reasonable indications for the application of ultraviolet light:

- skin disorders such as acne, psoriasis, boils, and so forth
- skin infections
- herpes zoster
- osteomalacia
- ulcers
- impetigo
- scleroderma

Contraindications

The following conditions and symptoms are considered reasonable contra-indications for the application of ultraviolet light:

- tuberculosis
- adrenal insufficiency
- burns
- diabetes mellitus
- eczema
- heart and liver disease
- herpes simplex
- hyperthyroidism
- keratosis
- keloids
- systemic lupus erythematosus (SLE)
- tumors
- photosensitive medications
- kidney disorders
- scleroderma

Summary

Each one of the modalities presented in this chapter exerts its primary effect on the superficial tissues of the body. Although many of the modalities presented are commonly used, both in clinical practice and as home therapy, none of these should be considered a primary treatment modality. It is important to understand that the use of such modalities should be considered adjunctive or supportive to more effective treatment methods. In addition, prolonged or habitual use of such modalities, either as home care or as a routine part of any chiropractic treatment, probably is not productive and should be avoided.

References and Suggested Reading

Prentice WE. Therapeutic modalities in sports medicine. St. Louis: Times Mirror Mosby, 1986.

Travell JG, Simons DG. Myofascial pain and dysfunction: the trigger point manual. Baltimore: Williams and Wilkins, 1983.

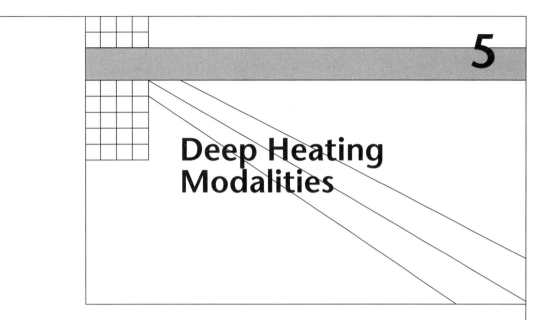

5

Deep Heating Modalities

Learning Objectives

At the completion of this chapter, you should be able to:

1. Describe the apparatus used to produce therapeutic ultrasound.
2. Describe the physiologic effects of ultrasound.
3. Describe the application techniques for using ultrasound.
4. Provide parameters for effectively using ultrasound.
5. List the indications, contraindications, and precautions for ultrasound use.
6. Describe the process of phonophoresis providing examples of chemicals that are used.
7. Describe the apparatus used to produce shortwave and microwave diathermy.
8. Describe the physiologic effects of diathermy.
9. Describe the application techniques for using diathermy.
10. Provide parameters for effectively using diathermy.
11. List the indications, contraindications, and precautions for diathermy.

The therapeutic application of heat directed at the deeper, subdermal tissues has been widespread for many years. The deep-heating agents can be broadly divided into two main categories: (1) those produced by the application of high-frequency sound vibrations (ultrasound) and (2) those produced by some type of electromagnetic energy (the diathermies). The use of therapeutic ultrasound is discussed in the first section of this chapter followed by a discussion of shortwave and microwave diathermy.

Ultrasound

The use of ultrasound waves for therapeutic purposes is extremely common in chiropractic practice. In fact, therapeutic ultrasound is one of the most widely used of all the passive modalities. It is used to treat a variety of disorders ranging from pain and inflammation to calcific bursitis and bone spurs. Although ultrasound is used frequently, it is, perhaps, the least understood and the most frequently abused modality.

Therapeutic ultrasound consists of sonic (**acoustic**) energy at a frequency of approximately 1.1 MHz—well beyond the normal range of audible sound waves. Many of the newer ultrasound units use an additional frequency range of 3.3 MHz. This higher frequency allows ultrasound to be applied in areas that previously were not sonated, such as the temporomandibular joint.

Ultrasound energy is produced by a process involving the conversion of electrical energy into mechanical energy in the form of sound waves. This is accomplished by passing an electrical current through a crystal, either **quartz** or **lead-zirconium-titanate (PZT)**. The electrical current causes the crystal to alternately expand and contract. The resulting expansion and contraction of the crystal transforms the electrical energy into mechanical energy in the form of sound waves, a process known as the "piezoelectric effect." The resulting mechanical vibration passes into the target tissue and creates a molecular vibration. This vibration creates friction between the molecules and the mechanical sonic energy is converted once again into thermal energy, which results in heating of the deeper tissues.

The therapeutic effect of ultrasound varies among various tissues. Ultrasound waves have an affinity for tissues that are highly organized, such as the tendons and ligaments. Consequently, these structures are selectively heated, whereas other less organized structures are affected to a lesser degree. Those tissues containing a high water content, such as fat and muscle, are not significantly warmed by the ultrasound waves. Other tissues, such as the periosteum, may be adversely affected by an accumulation of ultrasonic energy.

Apparatus

The ultrasound machine is a relatively simple device that has not changed much since its inception. The components of a therapeutic ultrasound unit (Figure 5.1) include:

- a power source
- a high frequency generator
- a transducer containing a piezoelectric crystal

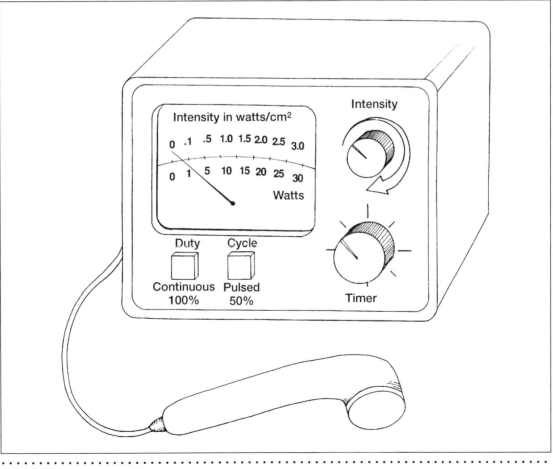

FIGURE 5.1   Components of the ultrasound unit.

Ultrasonic Energy

Conduction of the Sound Wave

Unlike sound waves that are found in the audible range, the energy produced by the ultrasound unit does not pass readily through air. To transmit the energy into the tissues of the body, some type of fluid material must be used between the sound head and the body. This fluid material is referred to as a **coupling agent**. The coupling agent may be some type of commercially available gel such as **Sonigel** or it may be water. In some cases an ice bag may be used to couple the sound head to the patient.

Note: It is important to recognize that the therapeutic effects of ultrasound are compromised if the transducer is not properly coupled to the skin. In addition, prolonged periods with inadequate coupling may seriously affect the integrity of the crystal and shorten the life of the ultrasound unit. To minimize these problems, many of the newer ultrasound units have sensing devices in the transducer that detect when the contact is not adequate and stop the flow of current to the crystal.

Penetration

Ultrasound waves are generally thought to penetrate as deep as 4 to 6 cm into the tissues (Figure 5.2). As stated, tissues with a high fluid content, such as blood and muscle, transmit sound waves much better than less hydrated tissues. The energy is best absorbed in tissues that are highly organized, particularly the ligaments and tendons, which makes ultrasound very beneficial in treating injuries to these areas.

Types of Waves

There are two types of sound waves produced: (1) a longitudinal wave and (2) a transverse wave (Figure 5.3). The longitudinal wave is emitted parallel to the direction of sound propagation. These waves are produced in all types of tissues. In contrast, the transverse waves are emitted perpendicular to the direction of wave propagation. These waves are only transmitted in solid substances and not in liquids or gases.

The longitudinal wave appears to be reflected at a rate of approximately 35% when it strikes the bone and is thought to reverberate between the surface of the bone and the underside of the periosteum (Figure 5.4). As a result, the soft tissue in the proximity of the bone receives an exaggerated effect caused by a rebound phenomenon. This is one of the primary hazards of therapeutic ultrasound and may result in periosteal burns if appropriate precautions are not taken. It is recommended that the ultrasound head be maintained in constant motion throughout the application to minimize this effect.

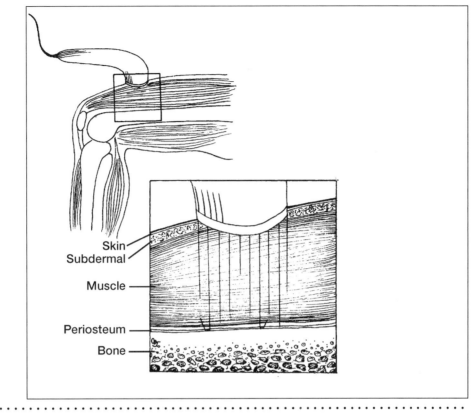

FIGURE 5.2   Ultrasound wave penetration is beneficial in treating injuries to the deeper tissues.

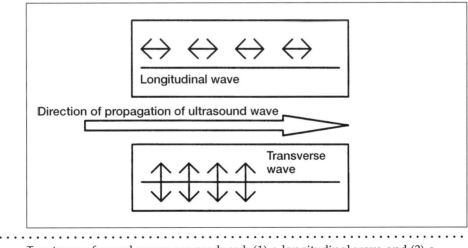

FIGURE 5.3   Two types of sound waves are produced: (1) a longitudinal wave and (2) a transverse wave.

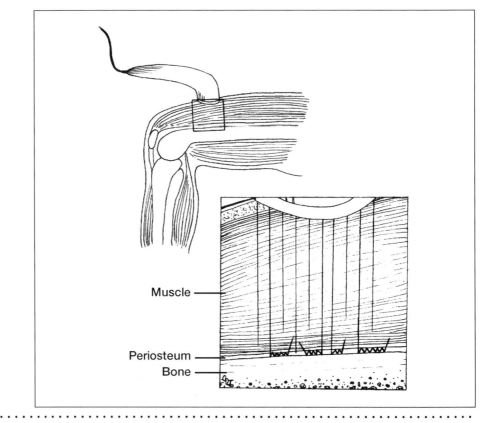

FIGURE 5.4   Ultrasound may result in burns to the periosteum.

Physiologic Reaction to Therapeutic Ultrasound

Therapeutic ultrasound is generally considered to be a form of deep heat. As such, the reaction of tissue to sonation is similar to that for any other form of deep-heating modality. These effects include: an increase in tissue temperature and in local metabolism, a softening of tissues, and an increase in local circulation. However, in addition to its known heating effects, ultrasound also produces several **nonthermal effects**, such as:

1. **Chemical reactions**—ultrasound vibrations stimulate the rate of chemical activity in the tissues, much like shaking a test tube in a laboratory.
2. **Biologic reactions**—ultrasound alters the permeability of the cell membrane, thereby enhancing the transfer of fluids and nutrients to the cells. There is some evidence that ultrasound may increase the rate of healing of certain injuries, which it is postulated may occur through this biologic response.

3. **Mechanical reactions**—the high-frequency vibration of ultrasound deforms the molecular structure of the tissues. If the intensity of the sound waves is great enough, the tissues may actually be irreparably damaged, a process known as **cavitation**. Therapeutically, this reaction is useful for its sclerolytic effects. Ultrasound has been shown to reduce spasm, to increase range of motion that has been lessened by adhesions and fibrosis, and to break up calcific deposits. It has also been shown to increase the extensibility of tendons.

4. **Acoustic streaming**—a unidirectional movement in the tissues that pulsed ultrasound produces, which is particularly marked at the boundaries of the cells and organelles. It has been observed that streaming induces changes in diffusion rates and in membrane permeability, both of which could alter the rates of protein synthesis and affect tissue repair.

Clinical Application

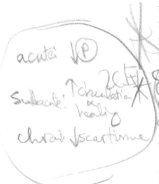

The ease with which it is applied, the high degree of patient comfort, and the relatively few complications that result from its use combine to make therapeutic ultrasound one of the most widely used passive modalities. It is used as a standard form of ancillary treatment for a wide variety of conditions in all stages of patient care. It may be used to control pain in the acute stage, to facilitate the healing process and improve circulation during the subacute stage, and to decrease scar tissue in later stages. Properly used, it is an extremely versatile modality to assist the clinician with a variety of clinical objectives. Improperly used, it is undoubtedly ineffective, although probably not harmful.

Patient Preparation

As with any treatment procedure, it is important to prepare the patient properly prior to any treatment with ultrasound. It is helpful to explain to the patient what the goals for treatment are and what can be expected both during and after treatment. In addition, the patient should understand the application technique and should be aware of any problems that might be encountered during treatment. Each patient should be questioned regarding any conditions that may contraindicate the use of ultrasound.

To apply therapeutic ultrasound, place the patient in a comfortable position and expose and clean the patient's skin. Remove any jewelry that might interfere with the application. Liberally apply a coupling agent to the area to be treated and also to the head of the transducer. It is a good idea to drape clean toweling over the patient's hair or clothing to avoid contact with the coupling agent. It may also be helpful to place a towel or blanket over any exposed skin to keep the patient warm.

Note: It is not uncommon for patients to ask about the difference between therapeutic ultrasound and diagnostic ultrasound. Diagnostic ultrasound differs in a number of significant ways. It uses a much different frequency that is not capable of any therapeutic heating. In addition, the application of diagnostic ultrasound is dependent on the image produced by the sound waves as they are reflected by various tissues.

Parameters

Intensity

The intensity of the ultrasound should be predetermined based on both the condition of the patient (acute, subacute, or chronic) and the thickness of the body part to be treated. The following guidelines are suggested:

- **acute condition/thin skin,** such as forearm or ankle, 0.5 to 1.0 w/cm² (watts per square centimeter)
- **acute condition/thick skin,** such as the thigh or buttocks, 1.0 to 1.5 w/cm²
- **chronic condition/thin skin,** 1.0 to 1.5 w/cm²
- **chronic condition/thick skin,** 1.5 to 2.0 w/cm²

Ultrasound sometimes is used to treat thin or bony areas such as the wrist and ankle by immersing both the body part and the ultrasound head in water. When ultrasound is applied using an underwater technique, it is suggested that approximately 0.5 w/cm² be added to the above parameters.

Note: My experience during many years of teaching physical therapy to doctors and assistants is that many individuals misunderstand and misuse ultrasound. It is important for the therapist to appreciate that the patient does not need to feel any sensation during the application of therapeutic ultrasound. Rather, it is essentially devoid of patient feedback unless it is used in combination with electrical stimulation, as will be described later. Too many therapists are instructed to "turn up the sound as high as the patient can tolerate." In some instances the patient may feel a slight warming of the transducer head as the treatment progresses, but under no circumstances should a patient feel any pain or intense heat.

Note: The intensity of the sound waves is not consistent over the entire surface of the transducer head (Figure 5.5). Rather, it contains areas of high and low intensity. The intensity is an average value per square centimeter of surface area of the sound head (**w/cm²**). One of the reasons that the sound head must be continually moved during the treatment is to average the overall application of sonic energy and avoid any "hot spots" that might otherwise harm the patient.

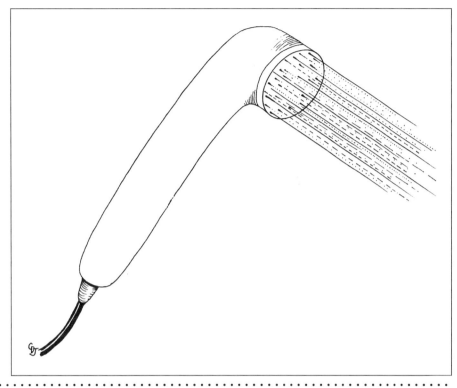

FIGURE 5.5   The ultrasound head contains areas of high and low intensity.

Duty Cycle

Ultrasound can be used as a deep heating therapy when the benefits of heat are desired. With this duty cycle, electrical energy is constantly directed through the crystal and ultrasonic energy is continuously produced, which heats the deeper tissues. This type of application is used most often during the treatment of a chronic condition, such as a myofascitis, or fibrous tissue and adhesions.

When heat is not desired, such as during the acute phase of an inflammatory condition, ultrasound can be modified in such a way that there is little or no accumulation of heat in the tissues. To minimize heat gain and to maximize the nonthermal effects of ultrasound, the **pulsed duty cycle** is used (Figure 5.6). In this setting, the generation and transmission of ultrasonic waves occurs intermittently during the course of the treatment. For instance, with a pulsed duty cycle of 50%, ultrasound is emitted for a period of 5 microseconds followed by a period of 5 microseconds during which no sound waves are produced. This alternating **on-off** cycle is repeated continually during the course of treatment. During the time that ultrasound is generated, heat is produced. However, during the time that the ultrasound is turned off, the body is

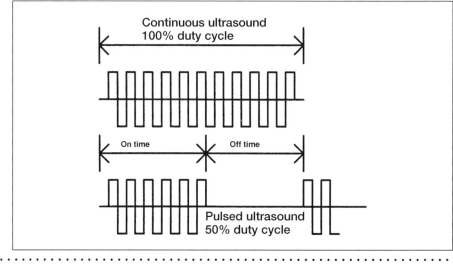

FIGURE 5.6   Pulsed duty cycle reduces the amount of heat produced.

able to dissipate the energy through the vascular supply to the area. Consequently, there is no appreciable heat gain in the tissues.

Note: Most manufacturers of modern ultrasound units provide several pulsed duty cycle settings. It is common to include a 50% cycle and a 30% or 20% cycle. The choice of which pulsed setting to use should be made based on the acuteness of the condition. Generally speaking, the more intense and painful the condition, the less intense the treatment.

Treatment Duration

There is a great deal of variation regarding the amount of time that is required for the application of therapeutic ultrasound. By convention, many therapists use times of 10 to 15 minutes. It is generally agreed, however, that much of the benefit derived from the application of this modality occurs in the first few minutes and, although not harmful, applications in excess of 7 or 8 minutes probably are unnecessary. The following guidelines are suggested as reasonable parameters:

- acute condition—4 to 6 minutes
- chronic condition—6 to 8 minutes

Note: Recent evidence suggests reducing all of the parameters for applying therapeutic ultrasound. It is suggested that applications of 0.5 to 1.0 w/cm^2 and 2 to 3 minutes may be adequate for many conditions and that greater intensities or longer treatment times are unnecessary. I am personally convinced that the following rule applies for all therapy: **When in doubt, use less.**

Application Technique

During the course of the ultrasound application the therapist should keep the sound head in firm contact with the patient. Failure to do so can damage the crystal and shorten the life of the transducer. The sound head should be continually moved slowly over the target tissue in overlapping concentric circles or longitudinal strokes during the course of treatment. It should not be allowed to remain in one place, as this may focus the energy in a small area and increase the risk of periosteal burns. The effect is like holding a magnifying glass over a pile of kindling; when the glass is held at just the right angle to the sun, the resulting solar energy produces enough energy to start a fire. Even a little movement of the magnifying glass reduces the energy from the sun and makes it impossible to start a fire (Figure 5.7).

Underwater Application

The contour of some areas of the body, such as the hands, wrists, and ankles, are not conducive to the application of ultrasound by the common inflexible type of sound head. In addition, the tissue of many of these areas are so thin that the underlying bone is too close to the surface for a safe application. As a result, a common modification is to use ultrasound underwater. To accomplish this, the body part to be treated is immersed in a container of warm water (Figure 5.8). The sound head is immersed in the water and directed at the target while being held at a safe distance, approximately 1 to 2 inches away. As with the typical ultrasound treatment, the sound head is moved slowly and continuously during the course of the treatment. The parameters are adapted by increasing the intensity of the sound as described above.

Note: Most patients will experience a greater sensation when ultrasound is used with the underwater application technique.

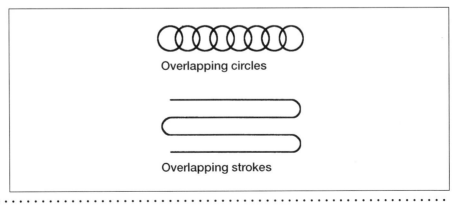

Overlapping circles

Overlapping strokes

FIGURE 5.7   Sound head should be moved in concentric circles or longitudinal strokes continually during the course of treatment to decrease the risk of periosteal burns.

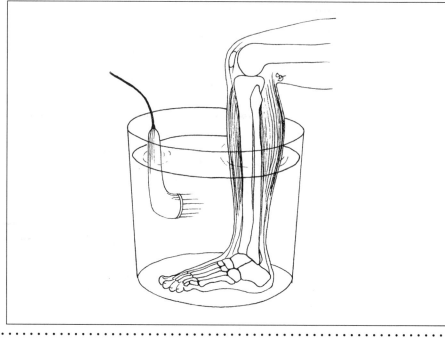

FIGURE 5.8   Underwater ultrasound technique.

Ultrasound can also be applied underwater with a slight modification of the above technique. In this application, the sound head is placed underwater, as described, but it is directed away from the target tissue and toward the sides of the container (see Figure 5.8). It is allowed to remain stationary throughout the course of the treatment as long as it is directed away from the tissue.

An effective method of applying ultrasound during the acute stage of injury involves immersing the injured part (*e.g.*, sprained ankle) in a bucket of ice water. The combination of ice water immersion and underwater pulsed ultrasound can have a dramatic effect on edema and pain following an acute injury.

Combined Ultrasound Electrical Stimulation

One of the more frequently used and useful modifications of therapeutic ultrasound involves combining it with electrical stimulation (Figure 5.9). This is accomplished by simultaneously directing both sound waves and electrical current through the transducer head. In addition to emitting acoustic energy, the sound head becomes the **active electrode** in an electrical stimulator (see section on electrical stimulation). The combined effect of these two modalities allows the therapist to warm the deeper tissues, to improve cellular transport mechanisms, to soften connective tissues, and generally to improve circulation with the ultrasound. At the same time, the

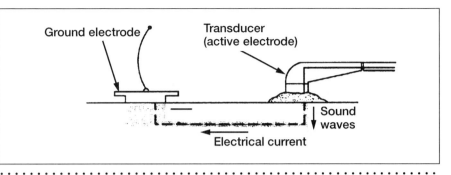

Ground electrode

Transducer
(active electrode)

Sound
waves

Electrical current

FIGURE 5.9   Ultrasound often is used in combination with electrical stimulation.

electrical stimulation reduces pain by closing the pain gate and it improves muscle tone, function, and circulation by producing muscle contraction. This has a dramatic effect on many chronic conditions such as myofascial trigger points and has the added advantage of significant patient awareness.

Clinical Application

As stated, it is helpful to explain the treatment to the patient prior to any application. Although patients do not feel ultrasound, they do feel a tingling sensation or "pins and needles" that results from the electrical current. In addition, if the intensity of the electrical stimulation is adequate, they will experience muscle twitching. Some patients respond better to ultrasound when they "feel" some sensation.

Note: Some patients who have been treated previously with this combination of ultrasound and electrical stimulation who were not adequately informed about the effects of the modalities, may associate the tingling sensation with the ultrasound.

Patient Preparation

The patient should be prepared as for the application of therapeutic ultrasound described above. In addition, the application of electrical stimulation requires the use of at least two electrodes. As previously described, the transducer head of the ultrasound becomes the **active electrode** of the electrical stimulating device. A second electrode, the **dispersive** or **ground electrode**, must also be connected to the patient. This second electrode often consists of a large 8 × 10 inch pad, but smaller pads may be more convenient to use. The dispersive electrode should be placed on the patient in some convenient location, such as the lower back or under the thigh. Some type of moist barrier, either a moistened sponge or an electrical gel must be placed between the electrode and the skin. (Refer to the section on electrical stimulation for further explanation of electrode placement.)

Note: It is important to note that the dispersive electrode should **NOT** be placed in such a manner that the electrical current passes through either the chest or the abdomen. For example, if the tissue to be treated is the lumbar paraspinal muscles, the pad should **NOT** go under the patient's abdomen.

Combination Ultrasound Settings
The parameters for the ultrasound component should follow the same guidelines listed in the previous section and should be based on both the acuteness of the condition and the thickness of the body part to be treated.

Combination Electrical Stimulation Settings
With this type of application of electrical current there are only two settings that are modified: (1) the **pulse frequency** and (2) the **intensity.** (For a detailed explanation of these settings, see the section on electrical stimulation.) The **pulse frequency** should be set at a relatively high rate of **80 to 100 Hz.** The **intensity** should be raised gradually to a gentle muscle contraction or **motor level stimulus (MLS)**. As with other forms of electrical stimulus, it is often desirable to increase the intensity gently during the course of treatment as the patient adapts to the sensation.

   Note: It is not clinically important whether the ultrasound or the electrical portion is selected first. However, it is suggested that the electrical current be established prior to raising the intensity of the ultrasound, which eliminates the need to move the sound head while setting the intensity of the electrical stimulation.

   The combination of ultrasound and electrical stimulation is often used to treat myofascial trigger points. The combined effect derived from the warming produced by the ultrasound and the analgesic effect of the electrical stimulator render the muscle containing the trigger point pliable. It is helpful to stretch the muscle following the treatment while it is warm and flexible.

Phonophoresis
In addition to its biologic and thermal effects, ultrasound may be used to drive various substances into the subcutaneous tissues. It has been suggested that this process allows the transfer of chemicals, such as analgesics and anti-inflammatory agents, to a depth of approximately 1 to 2 mm. This may provide a more local application of medications than oral ingestion and may minimize any systemic side effects that might otherwise occur. The use of ultrasound waves to introduce substances into the body through the skin is termed "phonophoresis."

   Technique. The technique for phonophoresis is essentially the same as for the standard application of therapeutic ultrasound. Instead of using an inert substance, such as the coupling agent, a variety of ointments containing chemicals, such as hydrocortisone, are used. The solution is massaged into the skin over the target area prior to sonation. Sonation parameters are the same as those listed above for ultrasound in general.

The selection of particular chemical substances is based on the condition and on the known physiologic response of the chemicals. It should be noted that phonophoresis does not lend itself to underwater applications.

Note: Because the practice of chiropractic does not include the use of materia medica, chiropractors using phonophoresis should check their local state guidelines and practice act to ensure that any chemicals used fall within their particular scope of practice.

Phonophoresis Chemicals. The following chemical substances are used with ultrasound:

- **hydrocortisone**—available over the counter in 1% solutions; typically used as an anti-inflammatory agent and may provide some analgesia.

- **mecholyl**—provided as an ointment with 0.025% methacholine and 10% salicylate; an effective vasodilator that is suggested for a variety of vascular conditions and neurovascular deficits.

- **lidocaine**—available as a 5% ointment (Xylocaine); used primarily as an analgesic in acute conditions.

- **iodine**—available over the counter in ointment form combined with methyl salicylate (Iodex); used as a vasodilator, as an anti-inflammatory, and as a sclerolytic agent in cases of scars, fibrosis, and adhesions.

- **salicylate**—available over the counter in a 10% ointment (Myoflex); used as an anti-inflammatory agent.

- **zinc**—available over the counter as a 20% ointment of zinc oxide; contributes to the healing process and is used to treat open wounds and lesions.

Precautions

The safe application of therapeutic ultrasound requires an understanding of the potential deleterious effects, such as periosteal burns and tissue cavitation. Consequently, the therapist should heed the following precautions:

- maintain continual motion of the sound head during the entire treatment.

- maintain proper lubrication of the patient. Because some of the coupling agent may be absorbed into the skin, it may be necessary to use additional coupling agent as the treatment proceeds.

- avoid using ultrasound over bony prominences, such as the spinous processes or acromion process. It is not uncommon to use ultrasound bilaterally on patients with lower back pain. Under such circumstances it is preferable to treat one side and then the other rather than moving the sound head from side to side.

• avoid using ultrasound directly over the spine.
• avoid using ultrasound over nerve plexuses or superficial nerves, such as the ulnar nerve.
• avoid using ultrasound over the carotid bodies or the anterior portion of the neck.

Indications

Ultrasound enjoys extremely wide use in clinical practice. The following conditions are considered reasonable indications for the application of therapeutic ultrasound:

• most acute or chronic musculoskeletal conditions, such as myositis, fibrositis, capsulitis, bursitis, tendinitis, and so forth
• myofascial trigger points
• muscle spasms
• neuralgia
• neuromas
• calcific deposits
• osteoarthritis
• radiculitis
• joint contractures

Contraindications

The following conditions are considered contraindications for the application of therapeutic ultrasound:

• infection
• peripheral vascular disorders
• peripheral neuropathies
• malignancies
• over metal implants
• over epiphyseal plates of growing children
• over gravid uterus
• for patients on blood thinning medication
• over bony prominences
• over nerve plexuses
• near a pacemaker
• over the eyes, heart, reproductive organs, or brain

Diathermy

The term diathermy means **deep heat**. Referring to the electromagnetic spectrum, currents with oscillations greater than 10,000 Hz are called "high frequency currents" (see Fig. 4.1). Both **shortwave** and **microwave diathermy** are grouped in this category. The currents produced by each of these modalities are used specifically to produce heat in the deeper tissues. Shortwave diathermy uses frequencies of 13.56 MHz and 27.12 MHz. The energy used by shortwave diathermy exists in a range that is very close to that used by commercial radio and television stations. Consequently, the frequency is regulated by the Federal Communications Commission (FCC). Microwave diathermy uses frequencies of 915 MHz and 2450 MHz.

Shortwave Diathermy

Shortwave diathermy has been used for many years. Although it is one of the most commonly applied physical modalities currently in use, it is perhaps one of the least understood. It is also one of the few modalities that is used for many conditions other than musculoskeletal aches and pains (*e.g.*, bronchitis, prostatitis, and sinusitis).

The application of shortwave diathermy involves the production of a high-frequency electromagnetic field in which both the patient and the diathermy apparatus are placed. The frequency most often used is 27.12 MHz with a wavelength of 11 m. The energy created by this field causes ions in the tissues to vibrate. This vibration is **converted** to heat in the deep tissues of the body.

Apparatus

The components of a shortwave diathermy unit (Figure 5.10) include:

- power supply
- direct current
- an oscillator that produces the high-frequency current
- power amplifier
- patient tuning circuit with applicators that allow energy to be transferred to the patient

Applicators

There are two types of treatment applicators (electrodes) used in shortwave diathermy: (1) condenser, and (2) inductor. The condenser applicators (also known as capacitors) provide an energy field that is mostly electrical, whereas the inductor type primarily provides a magnetic field.

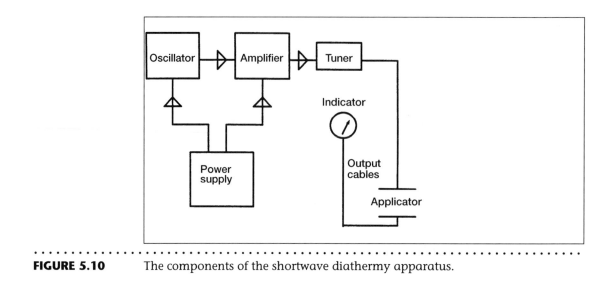

FIGURE 5.10   The components of the shortwave diathermy apparatus.

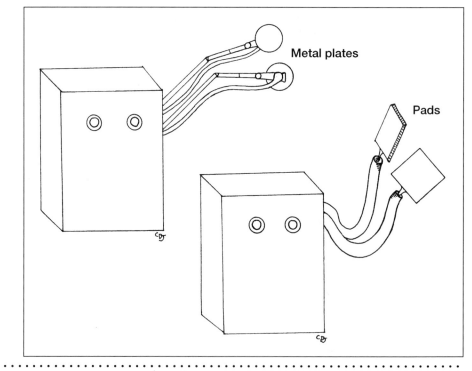

FIGURE 5.11   Condenser field applicator uses two separate pads or metal plates with an air-
                     space between them.

The **condenser field** applicator uses two separate pads or metal plates with an airspace between them (Figure 5.11). The current passes from one plate to the other, and both the air and the patient's tissues become part of the electric field and function as the dielectric between the two electrodes. The heat is strongest near the electrodes where the density of the field is the greatest.

The pads are placed directly on the patient with a single layer of toweling on the skin to absorb moisture. The metal plates are placed at a distance of 2 to 3 cm from the skin, with an airspace between the plates and the patient. The electric field produced by condenser-type applicators is absorbed readily by the skin and subcutaneous fat, and there may be considerable build-up of heat in the superficial tissues. Consequently, this type of shortwave diathermy is less helpful when treating tissues with overlying layers of fat. The tissues that are good conductors, such as muscles and blood, will receive the greatest heating effect.

The **inductive field** applicator is usually some type of drum, either a hinged drum or a single drum (Figure 5.12). Induction coils also are used

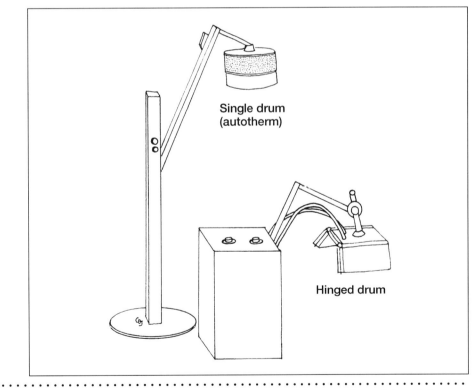

FIGURE 5.12   Inductive field applicator is usually some type of drum, either a hinged drum or a single drum.

with this method. The applicator is placed directly over the target area, which is covered by a single layer of toweling. The induction type of applicator produces a magnetic field that passes through the superficial tissues and is absorbed best in tissues with a high electrolyte content, such as muscle and blood. It is, therefore, the preferred method for heating the deep layers of muscle.

Circuit Resonance

To use shortwave diathermy effectively the unit must be **in tune** with the patient. Because the electromagnetic field surrounding each patient is slightly different and because the patient and the apparatus become part of the same circuit, the apparatus must be adjusted for each patient. This is similar to tuning a particular frequency on a radio to select a given station.

A simple demonstration to illustrate this *tuning* effect is as follows:

1. Turn on the shortwave diathermy and allow it to warm up.
2. Place an incandescent light bulb in the vicinity of the diathermy unit.
3. Move the light bulb toward the unit and away from the unit and observe the intensity of the light emitted. As the bulb comes in contact with the electromagnetic field, it will glow. The more *in tune* the bulb is with the field, the brighter the light emitted.

Pulsed Diathermy

Many manufacturers of diathermy units provide a **pulsed** mode, believing that the pulsations reduce the amount of heat generated. It is claimed that this nonthermal method of applying shortwave diathermy yields a variety of therapeutic effects that are somehow different. The current literature does not support this contention, and there does not appear to be any specific advantage in using pulsed diathermy.

Physiologic Reaction

As with other heating devices, the application of heat to the tissues of the body creates a variety of effects. The following have been noted with shortwave diathermy:

- increase in tissue temperature
- increase in metabolic rate
- vasodilation and increase in circulation
- elevation of capillary pressure

- increased white blood cell activity
- enhanced removal of metabolic wastes
- relaxation of spastic muscles
- softening of connective tissues
- increased endocrine activity
- increased circulation in viscera

Clinical Application

Apparatus Selection

As stated, the type of shortwave applicator selected is made based on the type of tissue to be heated. Condenser (capacitor) types are best equipped to provide relatively superficial heat to a broad area of the body. Inductive types are best equipped to provide heat to the deeper tissues, particularly the muscle. In many instances, however, the selection is based more on the equipment available than on the specific condition.

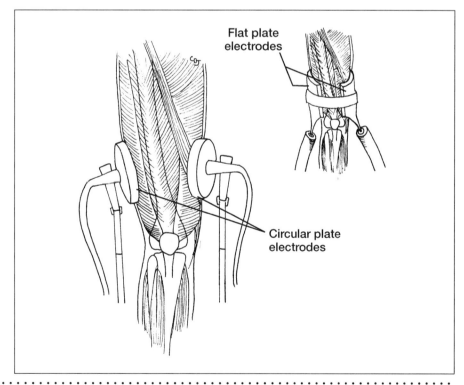

FIGURE 5.13   With the condenser type electrode, the tissue to be heated is placed directly between the two pads or plates.

Electrode Placement

If the electrodes used are condenser, place the tissue to be heated directly between the two pads or plates (Figure 5.13). The pads can be separated further to reduce the amount of heat applied. If the electrodes used are inductive, position the drum so that the part to be heated lies directly underneath the drum (if a single drum is used) or between the two wings (if a hinged drum is used). When using the induction-type pads, place them directly over the target tissue (Figure 5.14).

Regardless of the type of diathermy unit used, it is important to place a clean, dry towel on the skin under the electrodes. The towel will absorb any moisture that accumulates on the skin and will help to prevent burns. It is also important to remove any metal objects, such as belt buckles, glasses, earrings, or bra straps, that might be heated. Also, patients should remove contact lenses prior to shortwave diathermy applications.

Intensity

Although shortwave diathermy enjoys fairly widespread use, its application remains somewhat vague. There are no specific parameters or guidelines for adjusting the intensity of the shortwave diathermy unit. If the unit has an

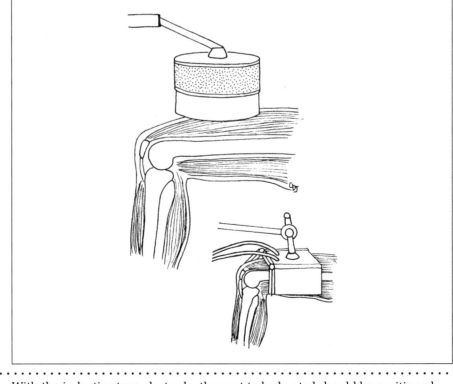

FIGURE 5.14   With the inductive type electrode, the part to be heated should be positioned directly underneath the drum.

automatic tuner, the suggestion is to raise the intensity until the patient feels a comfortable (never painful) sensation of general warming. Patients in pain should be treated at intensity levels slightly lower.

Tuning the Patient

As with the intensity setting, there are no clear guidelines regarding the "resonance" of the patient. Most units contain a control knob to adjust the machine to the patient's circuitry. With many older units, the resonance dial is set in the middle range of the indicator. Some of the newer equipment has meters or indicator lights that assist the operator in determining when the correct setting has been obtained. Some units automatically tune to the patient's resonance. The intensity of the machine is set using the following guidelines:

- If the unit has a manual tuner, the output dial is raised to one third of the total output. The tuner dial is adjusted to tune the patient circuit to the resonance of the unit. As the tuner is altered, the needle will rise and fall. It should be maintained at the highest available reading.
- If the unit has an automatic tuner, the output is set at a level that produces a gentle sensation of warming.

Treatment Duration

Treatment times vary between 10 and 30 minutes. The time is based on the condition and the patient. In general, as with most other forms of therapy, shorter, less intense treatments are used in the early stages of care and longer, more intense treatments are applied in the later stages. An application schedule of two times per week is considered safe for most conditions.

Indications

The following conditions and symptoms are considered reasonable indications for the application of shortwave diathermy:

- those conditions listed as indications for superficial heat
- sinusitis
- prostatitis
- otitis media
- bronchitis, chronic obstructive pulmonary disease (COPD), and other respiratory conditions
- pelvic inflammatory disease
- mastitis
- pleurisy
- dysmenorrhea

Contraindications

The following conditions and symptoms are considered contraindications for the application of shortwave diathermy:

- those conditions listed as contraindications for superficial heat
- acute inflammatory conditions or edema
- vascular conditions or hemorrhage
- tumors
- metal implants (including dental appliances and IUDs)
- malignancy
- menstruation
- pacemakers
- children or senile patients
- dressings or casts over injuries
- infections
- pregnancy
- over wet skin
- bleeding ulcers
- patients on anticoagulant therapy
- varicose veins
- thrombosis

Precautions

The following precautions should be observed during the use of shortwave diathermy:

- it should not be used at the same time as any other form of electrical modality.
- the patient should not be in contact with any metal objects and diathermy should not be used with a metal table.
- diathermy should NEVER be used near anyone who has an implanted pacemaker.
- the patient's skin should be checked periodically to ensure proper reaction to heat.
- avoid situations that might concentrate the energy in a particular area.

Microwave Diathermy

Microwave diathermy is similar to shortwave diathermy in its use as a deep heating modality. It is markedly different, however, in its mechanics and physics. The high-frequency energy produced by microwave units is directed or beamed toward the patient. This beaming allows the energy to be focused more on a given area than is possible with shortwave units.

The application of microwave diathermy involves the production of an electromagnetic field at a frequency of 2450 MHz. Heating is caused by friction produced by the vibration of molecules in the target tissue. As with condenser-type shortwave units, deep heating is difficult in the presence of subcutaneous fat.

Apparatus

The components of a microwave diathermy unit include:

- power supply
- magnetron oscillator that generates the high frequency wave
- treatment applicator (electrode)

Types of Applicators
Unlike shortwave diathermy, the energy produced by microwave units can be beamed at only one surface at a time. The target surface must be flat to reduce the amount of energy that is reflected. There are two types of applicators currently in use: (1) circular (diameter 4 to 6 inches) and, (2) rectangular (4.5 × 5 inches or 5 × 21 inches). The circular electrodes produce maximal output at the periphery of the field, whereas the rectangular electrodes produce the maximal output in the center of the field.

Physiologic Reaction

The reaction of the tissue to microwave heating is similar to that of shortwave units. The primary difference is the extent of the reaction as follows:

- tissue is heated much more locally.
- there is little penetration to organs (the depth of penetration is only about one third that of shortwave diathermy).
- there is little effect on circulation compared with shortwave diathermy.

Clinical Application

Treatment Electrode Selection
Selection of the appropriate treatment applicator is dependent on the shape of the field desired and on the target tissue's anatomy.

Electrode Placement
The electrode should be placed directly over the tissue to be heated at a pre-determined distance. This distance is based on the size of the applicator head; the manufacturer's directions should be followed precisely. It is not necessary to use a towel on the patient as with shortwave diathermy.

Intensity
As with other diathermy units, proper dosage is based on a subjective perception of gentle warming by the patient. The patient will feel a more localized heating with this type of diathermy.

Treatment Duration
Microwave treatments are generally slightly shorter than shortwave treatments, typically between 10 and 20 minutes, with times greater than 20 minutes inadvisable. It should be noted that the magnetron takes a considerable time to develop sufficient energy and should be given time to warm up prior to its application.

Indications

The indications for microwave diathermy are essentially the same as those listed for both shortwave diathermy and superficial heating agents. Microwave diathermy is preferred over shortwave diathermy when precision regarding the area to be heated is desired.

Contraindications

The contraindications for microwave diathermy are essentially the same as those listed for shortwave diathermy and superficial heating agents.

Precautions

The following precautions should be observed when applying microwave diathermy:

- avoid contact between applicator and skin.
- any perspiration should be wiped off skin as it develops.
- the patient and the operator should be provided with special wire mesh goggles to prevent damage to the lens.
- keep watches and hearing aids away from the unit.

Case 1: Ultrasound

Frank J., a 42-year-old grocer, presented with a primary complaint of lower back pain. His problem began approximately 2 days prior to the visit while he was carrying a heavy box at work. He states that he was carrying the box down several steps and slipped. He did not fall but felt that the misstep jarred his lower back. His pain is primarily located in the region of the right sacroiliac joint and he rates it as a 6 on a 0 to 10 scale. He admits to having several episodes of lower back pain in the past but none quite as painful as this.

Evaluation reveals tenderness to palpation over the right sacroiliac joint and right gluteal muscles. Range of motion of the lumbar spine is reduced in flexion and left side bending. Straight leg raising produces some mild pain on the right side when raised to 90 degrees. The Faber test produces pain on the right side in the region of the right sacroiliac joint. Bilateral muscle strength, deep tendon reflexes, and sensation are normal. Standing Gillet test reveals some difficulty in raising the right leg. Motion palpation reveals (1) a reduction in range of motion of the right sacroiliac joint compared with the left and (2) a flexion and left lateral bending restriction at the L5-S1 joint.

Based on the information provided during the history and examination, you conclude that Frank has a moderate sacroiliac sprain. Because he has not had significant problems with his back in the past and is in generally good health, his prognosis is optimistic. A full recovery is anticipated within a few weeks. The treatment plan involves two primary objectives: (1) to relieve the pain and discomfort in the right sacroiliac joint and (2) to restore full function to the joint.

1. Pain relief—it is decided that pulsed ultrasound will be used to address the pain in the sacroiliac joint. Ultrasound has the advantage of both decreasing pain and improving circulation in the injured area. The following parameters are used:
   - duty cycle—pulsed
   - intensity—1.0 watts/cm²
   - time—5 minutes

2. Restore function—spinal manipulation is the treatment of choice to establish normal range of motion to both the sacroiliac joint and the L5-S1 articulation. A high velocity, low amplitude side posture manipulative procedure is selected for each restriction. Prior to manipulation, the sacroiliac joint is stretched manually in both flexion and extension ranges. Frank is provided with knee to chest exercises and instructed to perform 10 repetitions every 2 hours for the next few days. It should not be necessary for him to be placed on temporary disability from work and he is instructed to continue his work activities using the pain to guide his activities.

The initial treatment plan involves the application of both pulsed ultrasound and spinal manipulation on a daily basis for the first three days. A reassessment is planned at the time of the third visit. If adequate improvement is achieved in relieving pain and improving range of motion, ultrasound will be discontinued. It is expected that a 3- to 4-week course of manipulation on a twice weekly basis will be adequate to establish full range of motion of the lumbar spine and pelvis. As the condition improves, Frank will be provided with additional exercises and will be assigned to a back school program to teach him safe lifting techniques.

Case 2: Ultrasound/Electrical Stimulation Combination

Debbie R., a 38-year-old secretary, presents with a chronic history of low back and leg pain. She states that her problem began several years ago after a particularly long automobile trip. She has pain in the middle of the lower back at the level of L4-5, in the right gluteal region, and down the posterior aspect of the right thigh. She estimates the lower back pain to be 4 or 5 on a 0 to 10 scale and describes the pain as "sharp and electrical." It comes and goes with certain movements, especially backward bending. The gluteal pain is described as more like a toothache and is graded at 5 on the 0 to 10 scale. This pain is more constant and increases with prolonged sitting. The pain in the posterior thigh is described as a "hot sensation." It only comes when she is tired or has been on her feet for long periods. Debbie relates no history of problems prior to the automobile trip previously described. She states that the problem appears to be worsening and currently she is taking over-the-counter pain medication.

Examination reveals palpatory tenderness in the lower back on the right side of L4-5 with radiation of tenderness to the right gluteal region. Palpation of the right piriformis muscle produces extreme tenderness with pain referral to the right posterior thigh. The patient states that the thigh pain feels the same as that previously experienced. Straight leg raising is normal bilaterally with some shortening of the hamstrings noted. Faber test produces some discomfort in the right side. Thomas test produces some discomfort in the region of the right buttocks. Internal rotation of the right hip produces gluteal pain. Deep tendon reflexes and sensation are normal bilaterally. Motion palpation reveals restrictions in the lumbar spine at L4-5 and L5-S1 and in the right sacroiliac joint. In addition, compared to the left hip joint, the right is restricted.

It is determined that Debbie is suffering from several problems concurrently: (1) a piriformis syndrome, (2) intersegmental dysfunction in the lumbar spine, and (3) acetabular dysfunction. The treatment plan includes:

1. Piriformis syndrome—a combination of ultrasound and electrical stimulation is selected for treatment of the piriformis syndrome. The following parameters are used:

- electrical stimulation—80 Hz/motor level stimulus
- ultrasound—continuous duty cycle/1.5 watts/cm²/6 min

After the combination treatment, the piriformis muscle is stretched manually. Debbie is provided with a series of home stretching techniques for the piriformis muscle and is instructed to repeat the exercises at least four times each day.

2. Intersegmental dysfunction in the lumbar spine—manual manipulation of the spine is the preferred method of treatment for this component of the patient's condition. A series of manipulative treatments is recommended on a three times per week basis for the first 2 weeks.

3. Acetabular dysfunction—treatment of the acetabular joint restriction includes a combination of stretching procedures, mobilization, and manipulation. The exercises provided for the piriformis will also positively affect the hip joint.

Each treatment session will begin with the combination of ultrasound and electrical stimulation to the piriformis muscle. This will be followed with stretching of both the piriformis muscle and the hip joint. Mobilization of the hip joint will be used during the first two to three treatment sessions, at which point manipulation procedures will be added. Manipulation of the lumbar spine will begin with the first treatment and continue each time the patient is seen for the first 2 weeks. The patient will be re-evaluated after 2 weeks of treatment and necessary modifications made in the treatment program.

Case 3: Shortwave Diathermy

Jane B., a 35-year-old bank teller, presents with a chronic history of back pain and stiffness. She states that her back is sore most of the time and rates the pain at a 4 on a 0 to 10 scale. Periodically, the pain may intensify to 6 or 7. Her primary complaint is the stiffness that she feels in her back. She states that she feels 60 years old. There does not appear to be any injury or event that precipitated the problems.

Examination reveals a moderately overweight individual who is otherwise in good health. Palpation reveals bilateral tenderness in the lower thoracic and lumbar spine. Range of motion is markedly reduced throughout the lumbar spine and pelvis. Straight leg raising is limited to 60 degrees bilaterally with stretching of the hamstrings noted. Faber test reveals stiffness of both hip joints with some bilateral discomfort in the groin and sacroiliac joints. Deep tendon reflexes and sensation are normal bilaterally.

It is determined that Jane has a nonspecific low back pain and is diagnosed with chronic lumbago. In addition, she is generally deconditioned.

Because the pain appears to be related to the stiffness, the primary treatment objective is to restore range of motion to the spine and pelvis. The treatment regimen consists of shortwave diathermy followed by stretching, mobilization, and manipulation. Initially, treatment is to be three times weekly for the first 2 weeks. Jane will be provided with a home stretching program to perform twice daily. In addition, she is instructed to walk briskly each day. She is to begin with a 20-minute walk and gradually increase it to between 30 and 45 minutes. At re-evaluation treatment will be modified based on the degree of progress noted.

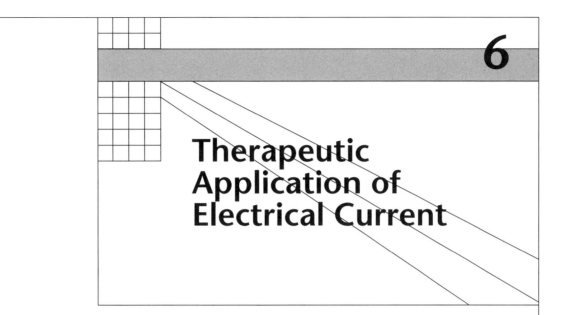

Therapeutic Application of Electrical Current

Learning Objectives

At the completion of this chapter, you should be able to:

1. Define electrical current.
2. Define:
   - amperes
   - volts and electromotive force
   - ohms
   - resistance and impedance
   - watts
   - conductor
3. Describe the physiologic response to electricity.
4. Differentiate between alternating and direct current.
5. Differentiate between a pulsed and a continuous (nonpulsed current).
6. Describe the various pulse parameters:
   - pulse shape
   - frequency
   - intensity
   - mode

- duration
- phase charge
- polarity
7. Describe the various types of electrodes used and list advantages and disadvantages of each.
8. Describe the electrode placement techniques.

The use of electrical current for medicinal purposes is not new. For many years it has been known that the introduction of an electrical current into the body produces a variety of effects, both positive and negative. Electric eels were used by ancient Egyptians and by Hippocrates. Scribonius Largus (Krusen, 1994) first recorded the use of electric eels for the treatment of headaches and gout. Much has been written about the use of electricity during the second half of the 18th century, but it took nearly 200 years before the therapeutic application of electrical currents became popular.

Basics

During the early years of electrotherapy, equipment was crude and application techniques were undoubtedly painful. Many of the underlying responses and physiologic mechanisms were not clearly understood. Recently, however, a great deal has been discovered about the mechanisms involved. Although many claims are made for the therapeutic application of electrical current, the nature and extent of the responses are dependent on two principal factors: (1) the particular physiologic response characteristics of the tissue affected by the current and (2) the nature of the current applied.

Principles of Electricity

To apply electrical current adequately in a clinical setting, it is important to understand some of the basic principles of electricity. **Electricity** is defined as "one of the fundamental forms of energy." **Electric current** consists of "the flow of electrons along some type of conducting medium." The **electrons** that make up the current are particles of matter possessing a negative charge. The total amount of electrical current is determined by the number of electrons and is measured in **amperes (amp)**.

Note: The amount of current in an electrical circuit in a typical house is usually less than 15 or 20 amp. Current in excess of this will "trip the breaker" and stop the flow of current. Typically, the current used in therapeutic electrical stimulators is described in **milliamperes (mA)**. Each milliampere is one thousandth of an ampere. The amount of current necessary to elicit a muscle contraction in most individuals is approximately 15 to 20 mA. Obviously, it does not take a great deal of electrical current to evoke a physiologic response.

As stated, electrical current is the flow of electrons along a conducting medium. For the electrons to flow, an electrical potential difference must exist between two points (Figure 6.1). The force that produces this flow of electrons is called the "electromotive force" (EMF) or the "voltage." Voltage is measured in **volts** and is defined as "the difference in electron population between two points."

Materials that allow the flow of electrons are termed "conductors." Water, for example, is an excellent conductor. Consequently, tissues with a high water or fluid content, such as muscles and fat, are good conductors. Other materials, such as wood and rubber, inhibit the flow of electrons; they are called "resistors." The resistance to current flow, also known as "impedance," is measured in **ohms.**

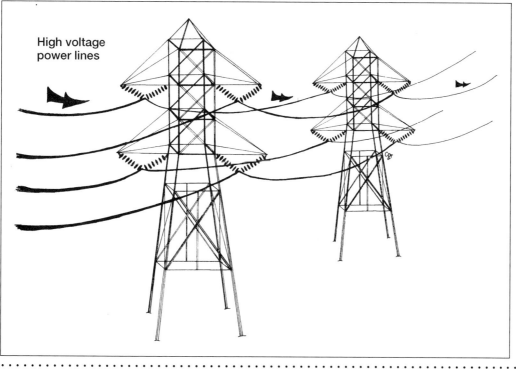

FIGURE 6.1   Electrical current flows along high tension wires because of the electrical potential difference that exists.

Note: The skin serves as a primary resistor to the flow of electricity. Skin resistance can be affected by a number of factors, such as dryness or dirt, hair, and skin oils. It is important to understand that the greater the resistance of the skin, the more current must be used to cross this physiologic barrier and the more uncomfortable the current becomes. One of the primary objectives in the design and manufacture of effective electrical stimulation devices is to overcome the natural resistance of the skin, which makes the introduction of electrical current more comfortable and acceptable to the patient. Various electrical modalities accomplish this in a number of different ways that will be discussed later in this text.

The flow of electrical current is directly related to the voltage and inversely related to the resistance. This relationship between current flow, voltage, and resistance is known as **Ohm's law** and is depicted by the formula:

current flow = voltage / resistance

(or $I = v / r$)

The amount of energy or power that is produced is determined by the number of electrons flowing (amperes) and the electromotive force (volts). This energy is measured in a unit called a **watt**.

watts = volts $\times$ amperes

To appreciate better the basic concepts of electricity we will compare electrical current to an x-ray beam (Figure 6.2). Because an electrical current and an x-ray are both forms of electromagnetic energy, they are affected by many of the same principles. The amount of radiation in the x-ray beam is measured by the number of electrons in the beam or the **milliamperes** multiplied by the time of exposure **(mA per second or MAS)**. Obviously, the greater the number of electrons, the stronger the x-ray and the greater its effect on the tissues in its path. The energy that drives the x-ray is the **kilovoltage** or the **KVP**. If greater penetration is desired, the energy of the x-ray beam must be increased. This is accomplished by increasing the KVP or the electrical potential difference.

The x-ray beam passes readily through the air (a conductor) until it enters the patient's body where it meets some resistance. Different tissues and materials resist to varying degrees. To overcome resistance, both the number of electrons (MAS) and the force driving the electrons (KVP) must increase. The effect that the x-ray beam has on the film is the result of this combination of electron numbers and electromotive force. In a similar manner, electrical current has an effect that is the result of both the number of electrons (mA) and the electromotive force (volts). The greater the number of electrons, the stronger the tissue response becomes. The

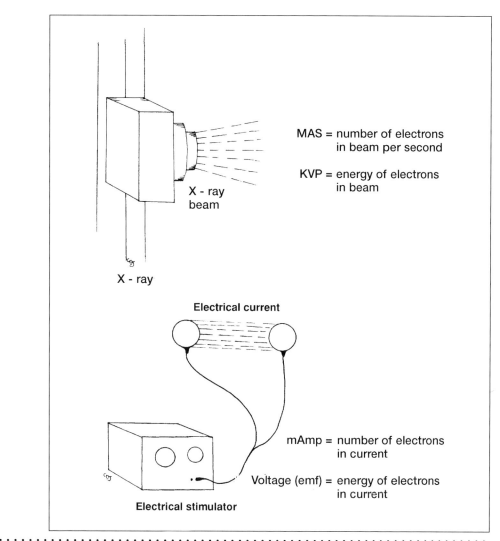

FIGURE 6.2   Comparision of x-ray and electrical circuit. Electrical current and x-ray are both forms of electromagnetic energy.

greater the electromotive force (emf), the deeper the penetration of the current.

Types of Electrical Current

Although there are a number of ways to classify electrical currents, there are only two principal types of current. These are differentiated by the direction of current flow (Figure 6.3).

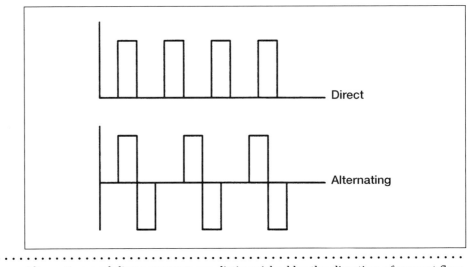

FIGURE 6.3   Alternating and direct currents are distinguished by the direction of current flow.

Direct Current (DC)

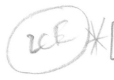

Electrons continually flow in the same direction with direct current. Because of this unidirectional flow, direct currents tend to align the electrons in their path. Consequently, they have a significant polarizing effect. This effect is utilized for certain therapeutic purposes such as iontophoresis. An example of a direct current is seen in the common 9 volt battery. Direct currents are also referred to as monophasic and have either a positive (+) or a negative (-) phase.

Alternating Current (AC)

With alternating current, the flow of electrons continually changes direction. Because the direction of current flow constantly reverses, the electrons are not allowed to align and there is no polarizing effect. An example of an alternating current is seen in the typical household electrical circuit. Alternating currents are also referred to as biphasic because they have both a positive and a negative phase.

Electrical current (both AC and DC) can also be differentiated based on the nature of its delivery. Current can be delivered in a steady stream of electrons (continuous) or in a series of electrical pulses (pulsatile) (Figure 6.4). Most currents are pulsed or pulsatile.

Continuous (Nonpulsed)

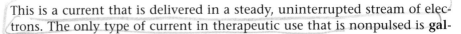

This is a current that is delivered in a steady, uninterrupted stream of electrons. The only type of current in therapeutic use that is nonpulsed is **gal-**

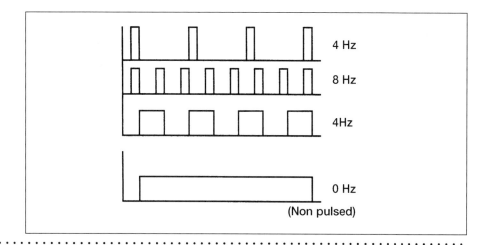

FIGURE 6.4   Electrical currents may also be desribed as continuous or pulsed currents.

vanic, which is a form of direct current. Galvanic current has limited clinical applications and exerts a very strong polarizing effect. It is a potentially
harmful current if used improperly. (Galvanic current is discussed under the
section on iontophoresis in Chapter 7.)

Pulsed (Pulsatile)

Most of the electrical stimulators currently in use (both AC and DC) deliver
a **pulsed** current. In other words, the current is delivered in a series of pulsations rather than a steady stream. By varying the parameters of the pulse,
we can elicit a number of different physiologic effects. Much of our discussion of the clinical application of electrical current focuses on modifications
of the pulse. By nature, pulsed currents have a much less polarizing effect
and are used in different ways than galvanic currents. They are not capable
of iontophoresis.

Physiologic Response

The application of electricity to the body involves a variety of physiologic
responses. These effects can be summarized in three basic areas:

Thermal Effects

The movement of an electrical current through a conductive medium produces a vibration of molecules. This vibration produces friction that leads to
an increase in temperature. Added to this vibration is natural skin impedance, which also leads to the production of heat. Although the thermal

effects are minimal with most therapeutic currents, they must be taken into consideration. Strong polarizing currents, such as galvanic, may cause serious burns if not used cautiously.

2) Chemical Effects

Electrical current produces the formation of new chemical compounds. The reaction to electrical current varies with the polarity of the electrode and, with some currents (*e.g.*, galvanic), this reaction can be significant. The production of potassium and sodium hydroxide under the electrodes of a galvanic current may lead to serious skin burns.

Physical Effects

In the clinical setting, electrical current typically is used for its physical effects. These physical effects can be divided into two areas:

Excitatory Effects

The most common application of electrical stimulation involves the effect that such currents have on the excitable tissues, particularly the peripheral nerve fibers. When an adequate stimulus (*i.e.*, a current that has sufficient intensity and duration) is applied to the tissues, the nerve is depolarized and an action potential is elicited (Figure 6.5). The resulting depolarization leads to sensory and motor responses that have predictable clinical uses. In fact, the vast majority of clinical applications involve the depolarization of sensory and motor nerves. Under certain circumstances, muscle fibers themselves may be excited by the electrical current. It should also be noted that, whereas not typically targeted by the clinician, the autonomic nerves are also affected by electrical current. This has affects on the body in ways that are not as well understood or as often utilized therapeutically.

Nonexcitatory Effects

As the electrical current passes through the body, an alteration in physiologic processes is seen. This alteration differs from tissue to tissue. Although all tissues are affected by the current, not all are excited. The effects, however, may be seen at several different levels: cellular, tissue, segmental, and systemic. These effects can be direct (*e.g.*, changes of cell membrane permeability) or indirect (*e.g.*, changes in blood flow). There is some evidence that electrical current may promote protein synthesis and stimulate tissue growth and repair. For example, electrical stimulation is often used to stimulate bone growth following spinal surgery. In addition, electrical stimulation is thought to affect both the ion-sensitive and voltage-sensitive channels in the cell membrane, thus enhancing intracellular transport

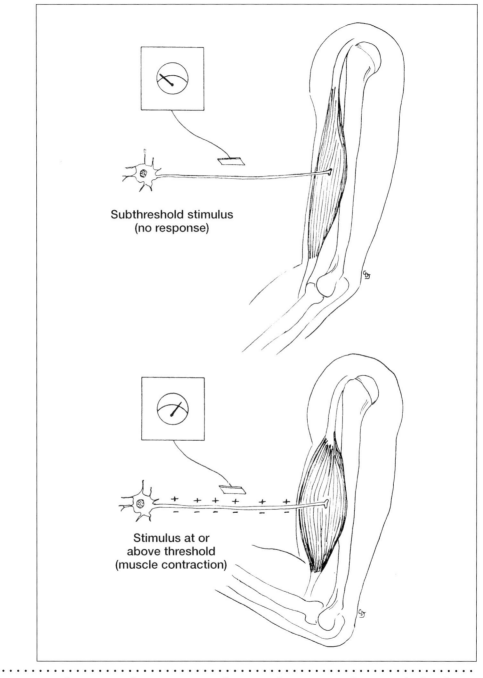

FIGURE 6.5 Depolarization of nerves occurs when an adequate stimulus is applied to the tissues.

mechanisms. At this point, there remain other physiologic responses that have yet to be identified and explained. It may be that once understood, the nonexcitatory responses to electrical current may offer new and exciting applications for this common therapy.

Pulsed Currents—Pulse Parameters

Electricity is a form of electromagnetic energy. Most electrical currents consist of a series of pulsations or pulses. With the exception of the true galvanic form of current, all of the electrical stimulators currently in use utilize a **pulsed** or **pulsatile** form of current. By altering the various parameters of the pulse, a number of different physiologic responses can be invoked. It is possible to modify the following parameters:

- shape of the pulse
- intensity of the pulse
- frequency of the pulse
- duration or width of the pulse
- mode of delivery of the current
- polarity
- pulse charge

To effectively administer any electrical stimulator in the clinical setting it is necessary to understand the effect each of these pulse parameters may have.

Pulse Shape

Each pulse of current has a particular shape or **waveform**. There are some unique waveforms that are used with specific types of electrical stimulators. For example, a high voltage generator (hvg) uses a double spike waveform that has a twin peak, whereas an interferential stimulator (ifc) uses a combination of sinusoidal waveforms. Great emphasis is often placed on the unique characteristics of particular pulse shapes. The manufacturers of electrical stimulation devices sometimes make claims that a particular stimulator is unique and different because of the dynamics of the pulse shape. Although there may be some truth in these claims, from a practical point of view the pulse shape is probably the least important parameter. Whenever a pulsatile electrical current is introduced through the skin, regardless of the type of current used, the resulting effect on the nerve fibers is essentially the same.

The pulse shape is important when considering patient comfort. Pulses with a gradual slope, such as the sinusoidal pulse, tend to be more comfortable than those with abrupt rises in current as seen with the square or rectangular wave. In addition, there may be instances when pulse shape is important from a physiologic perspective. The manufacturers of microcurrent stimulation devices claim that pulse shape is crucial at the cellular level. There is good rationale for this argument, however, many of these claims have yet to be substantiated.

The pulse shape (Figure 6.6) may be varied in any of the following ways:

- sine wave (sinusoidal)
- square wave
- twin-peaked wave
- asymmetric wave

Pulse Intensity

Intensity is a measure of the amount of electrical current available. Intensity is also called "amplitude" or "output" and is measured in **milliamperes (mA)**. Some of the newer electrical stimulation devices utilize a microamperage that is incapable of eliciting a neurologic response. These devices are thought to function by stimulating the cell membrane rather than the peripheral nerve.

Regardless of the type of electrical stimulation device used, as the intensity of the current is raised, the body responds in a predictable manner as follows:

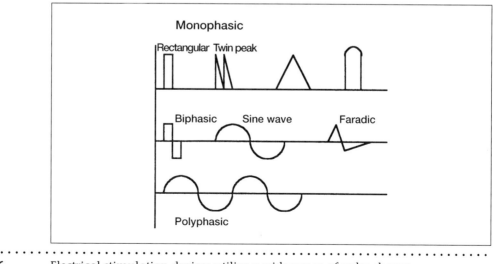

FIGURE 6.6 Electrical stimulation devices utilize a wide range of pulse shapes.

- At a level below **1 mA** there is not enough current to depolarize the nerve fibers and elicit any form of neurologic response. However, there does appear to be some evidence that such a **subthreshold stimulus** can produce a physiologic response. It is theorized that these low amplitude microcurrents affect the cell membrane permeability and may also affect cellular activity and growth. These small subthreshold currents are used by the **microcurrent stimulators (microamperage stimulation devices [MAS])**. Although many questions remain about the effectiveness of these devices, microamperage stimulation may be one of the most promising areas for future research in applying electrical stimulation.

- As the current intensity is increased, the threshold for depolarization of the large superficial sensory nerves is reached. This is perceived as a fine, tingling sensation by the patient that is similar to "pins and needles." It is referred to as a "sensory level stimulus" (SLS). This stimulation level is used for many pain control techniques, such as the classic TENS that target the superficial sensory nerves.

- As the current intensity is increased further, a stronger sensory stimulus is achieved. When the current reaches sufficient intensity to overcome the threshold of the motor nerves, these nerves also respond and a muscle contraction is experienced. This is referred to as a "motor level stimulus" (MLS). It should be emphasized that this motor level response does not replace any sensory effect that is achieved by stimulating the sensory nerves. Rather, it is a second response that is added to the first. The greater the amount of current at a motor level, the stronger the muscle contraction will become.

- Eventually, as the current intensity increases even further, the smaller, deeper C-fibers are stimulated. At this point the patient will experience a burning or aching type of pain that is referred to as a "noxious level stimulus" (NLS) or a **tolerable pain**. This uncomfortable stimulation level is used in several pain control techniques that may be helpful for chronic or resistant pain when other, less invasive methods have failed.

- Further increases in current intensity lead to an "intolerable pain" and eventually to tissue damage and necrosis.

Note: Intensity levels are determined prior to any stimulation and patients should be informed of exactly what they may expect. It is important to point out that, regardless of the intensity level required, all stimulation must be performed within the individual patient's ability to tolerate. A stimulation level that is acceptable for one patient may not be for another.

Note: It should be noted that the number of milliamperes necessary for this response varies widely from patient to patient. A number of factors influence the response, including type and size of electrodes, skin condition, hydration of the patient, and so forth. Consequently, when attempting to adjust an electrical stimulator to a specific intensity level, it is more important to watch the patient than the machine.

The physiologic effect of electrical current at varying intensities are as follows:

	Physiologic Effect
0-1 mA	imperceptible (subthreshold)
1-15 mA	tingling sensation to muscle contraction
15-100 mA	painful electrical shock
100-200 mA	cardiac or respiratory arrest
>200 mA	instant tissue burning

In addition to the level or amount of electrical current, there are several terms that should be understood when discussing current intensity (Figure 6.7):

- **Peak current**—this is the maximal amount of current delivered at the peak of the pulse. Whereas the peak current of most electrical stimulators is limited to approximately 50 mA, some stimulators such as HVG have an extremely high peak current, sometimes as much as 2500 mA.

- **Average current**—this is the average amount of current that is delivered during the stimulation. The lower the average current, the lower the risk of harm or discomfort to the patient. The average current is the result of an interaction between the peak current and the pulse width. The shorter the width of the pulse, the lower the average current will be. In nonpulsed galvanic current, the peak current and average current are equal.

- **Total current**—this is the total amount of current that is delivered during the stimulation. The greater the total current, the stronger the effect on the tissues.

Pulse Frequency

As with other forms of electromagnetic energy, frequency is defined as the number of pulses occurring in a 1-second period. Frequency is one of the most important variables for the various clinical applications of electricity. Pulse frequency is measured in **hertz (Hz)** and may also be referred to as "pulse rate, pulses per second (pps), cycles per second (cps), or rate."

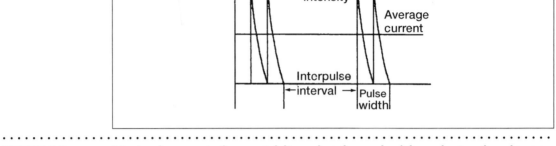

FIGURE 6.7   Maximal amount of current delivered at the peak of the pulse is referred to as the "peak current."

By varying both the intensity of the current and the frequency of the pulses, a number of different physiologic responses can be produced. The following frequencies are used at the intensity levels indicated:

Subthreshold Level Stimulus
The pulse rates used with microcurrent stimulation devices range from 0.5 per second to several hundred per second. It is suggested that lower pulse rates are preferable for chronic conditions and higher pulse rates for more acute conditions.

Sensory Level Stimulus (SLS)
80 to 100 Hz. At a sensory level, this high frequency produces a rapid stimulation of the large, superficial sensory nerves and effectively blocks the transmission of painful or noxious impulses. This is usually explained by using the pain gating mechanism of Melzack and Wall. By stimulating the sensory nerves at a high frequency, the current is said to "close the pain gate." This combination of high frequency and low intensity (sensory level) is used in the typical TENS type of treatment. It is referred to as "classic or high TENS."

5000 Hz. Such a frequency is also used to relieve pain, although not through the pain gating mechanism. It is thought that this high-frequency stimulus causes a rapid depolarization and repolarization of the nerve fiber that effectively blocks the conduction of the nerve impulse and thereby reduces pain. In some of the older literature this may be referred to as "Wedinsky inhibition." It is necessary to use a medium frequency stimulator for this type of stimulation as not all electrical stimulation devices are capable of such frequency ranges.

Motor Level Stimulus (MLS)
2 to 5 Hz. This low frequency rate is used to promote the release of endogenous pain-relieving chemicals such as beta-endorphin. It is used

with the electrical stimulation of acupuncture points and, in some patients, may produce long-lasting pain relief. It is referred to as "acupuncture-like TENS" or "LoTENS." The stronger the intensity of the current, the greater the effect appears to be. Unlike many other pain-relieving protocols that may respond to variations in parameters, the endorphin response appears to be dependent on using both low frequency and high intensity.

1 to 15 Hz. This frequency will elicit a nontetanizing muscle contraction or **twitch**. The slower the frequency of pulses, the more distinguishable each contraction becomes. These twitching contractions may be effectively employed to decrease edema and improve local circulation.

20 to 50 Hz. At a point usually between 15 and 20 Hz the individual muscle contractions become indistinguishable and a smooth **tetanizing** contraction is seen (Figure 6.8). This moderate frequency rate is said to produce **nonfatiguing tetany** and a **smooth** type of muscle contraction. Such contractions may be useful to increase range of motion, to decrease edema, and to decrease fibrous tissue and adhesions.

Above 50 Hz. A high-frequency rate greater than 50 Hz produces a **vigorous** type of muscle contraction that is referred to as a "fatiguing tetany." This particular frequency will elicit a strong muscle contraction and is used for reducing muscle spasms and for some muscle strengthening techniques.

Noxious Level Stimulus (NLS)

1 to 4 Hz. This frequency range may be combined with a noxious level current intensity to produce an electrical hyperstimulation analgesia. In addition to the low frequency and high intensity, this stimulation procedure uses small, pin-point electrodes. The physiologic mechanism of pain inhibiting pain is one of a counterirritant.

2 to 5 Hz. A low frequency rate is used to promote the release of beta-endorphins. Although this frequency range produces beta-endorphin release at a motor level intensity, the combination of low frequency and noxious intensity level will maximize this effect. With this protocol it is necessary for stimulation to last at least 20 minutes and not exceed 45 minutes.

70 to 100 Hz. This higher frequency range is used with a noxious level intensity and is referred to as "brief, intense TENS." This technique causes

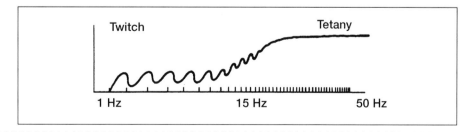

FIGURE 6.8   At a point between 15 and 20 Hz, individual muscle contractions become indistinguishable and a smooth contraction is seen.

fatigue in the sensory nerves and blocks the sensation of pain; a counterirritant effect is probably produced. This technique is particularly effective for treating chronic myofascial trigger points.

Note: The nervous system rapidly adapts or accommodates when it is exposed to a steady stimulus such as a constant frequency of 100 Hz. Consequently, the stimulus may tend to have a decreasing effect. Although this adaptation may be acceptable in some patients, it may be counterproductive in others. To minimize this adaptation of the nervous system, the current frequency may be changed or **modulated** during treatment. To accomplish this, the stimulator can be set to vary continually between two preselected frequencies (*e.g.,* 80-150 Hz). This is referred to as a "frequency sweep," a feature found on most modern electrical stimulators.

Duration of the Pulse (Pulse Width)

For a pulse of electrical current to elicit a neurologic response, it must have both adequate intensity and adequate time. Each pulse of current occupies a predetermined time from beginning to end. The width of the pulse is described as the length of time from the beginning of one pulse to the end of the same pulse and is measured in microseconds (Figure 6.9). The pulse width of most stimulators is approximately **250 microseconds** (usually set by the manufacturer). The wider the pulse, the greater the effect of the current. This is due to the fact that the current has more time to elicit a response. The interval between each pulse is referred to as the "interpulse interval" (Figure 6.10). The wider the interpulse interval, the lower the average current and the more comfortable the stimulation becomes.

Pulse width is related to the intensity of the stimulus as shown by the **strength-duration curve** (Figure 6.11). The longer the current is present, the lower the intensity necessary to produce a desired effect. When using a

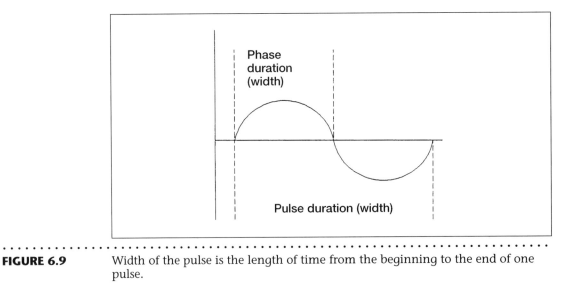

FIGURE 6.9   Width of the pulse is the length of time from the beginning to the end of one pulse.

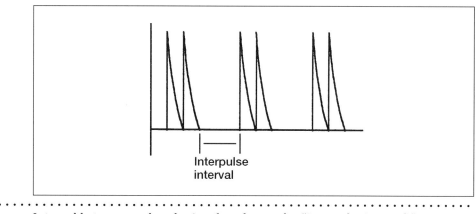

FIGURE 6.10 Interval between each pulse is referred to as the "interpulse interval."

wide pulse, it may only be necessary to use a small amount of current. However, because narrower pulses have less time to produce an effect, they require greater current intensities to elicit the same response.

When using a current with a narrow pulse width, the amount of current necessary to elicit a sensory response may be considerable. As seen in Figure 6.11, it takes a significant increase in current intensity to produce a motor response and even more to produce a noxious level current. This allows sufficient flexibility when attempting to target a specific nerve fiber—a process known as "discrimination." As the pulse widens, the ability to selectively discriminate each type of nerve fiber diminishes. In summary, the narrower the pulse width, the better the ability to discriminate

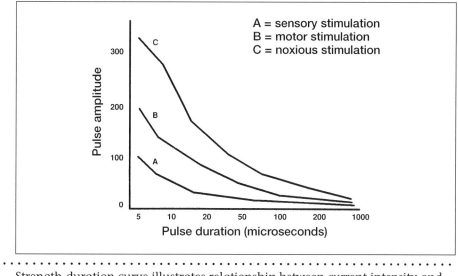

FIGURE 6.11 Strength-duration curve illustrates relationship between current intensity and pulse width.

(select a particular physiologic response) and the more comfortable the stimulation to the patient. The wider the pulse width, the stronger the stimulus. A narrow pulse width usually is preferred when patient comfort is required. A wider pulse width is useful when strong muscle contractions are needed.

Delivery Method (Mode)

The mode or method of delivery of the current is one of the more important parameters to be considered (Figure 6.12). Altering the mode enables the doctor to accomplish a variety of different therapeutic objectives. The current can be delivered in the following ways: (1) a **continuous current** is delivered in a steady, uninterrupted manner for the duration of the treatment (continuous currents are used for many pain control techniques, for decreasing edema, and to fatigue or relax tight muscles), and (2) an **interrupted current** is repeatedly turned ON and OFF at predetermined intervals throughout the course of the treatment. This interrupted current is sometimes referred to as a "surged" or a "pulsed" current. Two separate interrupted currents can be combined by connecting electrodes to antagonist muscles and alternating the ON and OFF cycles between the two currents. This is referred to as an "alternating" or "reciprocating" mode. These interrupted modes of delivering current are useful in creating intermittent muscle contractions to reduce edema, increase range of motion, and so forth. They may also help to reduce patient accommodation or adaptation to treatment.

The ratio of ON time to OFF time is dependent on the nature of the condition and may be varied as follows:

- during the acute phase of care the ON:OFF time should be relatively short, with a 1:1 ratio (*e.g.*, 5 seconds ON and 5 seconds OFF);

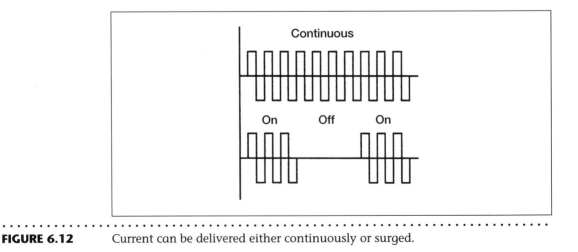

FIGURE 6.12   Current can be delivered either continuously or surged.

- as treatment progresses to the subacute phase, the ON:OFF time should be lengthened but the ratio remain the same 1:1 (*e.g.,* 10 seconds ON and 10 seconds OFF);
- during the later phases of treatment the OFF time should be lengthened and the ratio of ON:OFF time should be either 1:4 or 1:5 (*e.g.,* 10 seconds ON and 50 seconds OFF); during the OFF time the patient may be instructed to actively move or exercise the area being treated.

When an interrupted current is used, the intensity of the current is established at the beginning of the course of treatment. With each current interruption, the current is "ramped" when it comes ON again to allow for a gradual re-establishment of current (Figure 6.13). This current ramping makes the reintroduction of the interrupted current much more comfortable and tolerable to the patient and prevents any shocking or jolting that might otherwise occur. Many electrical stimulators have a preset current ramp that is automatically activated whenever an interrupted current is used. Some machines allow the clinician to control the ramp (both the rate of rise [ON] and the rate of decline [OFF]). For optimal effectiveness, the amount of time of the current ramp should not exceed one third of the total ON time of the current.

Polarity

When tissue is exposed to electrical current the ions in the tissue are aligned or polarized according to the direction of current flow. Under certain circumstances, such as that seen with galvanic current, this polarizing effect may be significant and may account for part or all of the physiologic response (*e.g.,* iontophoresis). However, the pulsed nature of most therapeutic electrical currents reduces the impact of any polarizing effect that might otherwise occur. For all practical purposes, with the exception of the low-

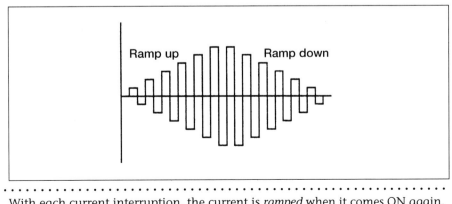

FIGURE 6.13   With each current interruption, the current is *ramped* when it comes ON again.

voltage galvanic current, the polarity of commonly used pulsatile currents is not significant. Consequently, polarity will not be considered at this point, but it will be discussed further in Chapter 7 dealing with iontophoresis. Because the direction of current flow in an alternating current (AC) is continually reversing, there is no polarizing effect in alternating current stimulators.

Pulse Charge

The pulse charge represents the accumulation of current in the tissues. The pulse charge is represented by the area under the pulse and is measured in **microcoulombs**. Alternating current has both a positive and a negative phase that effectively eliminates each other; consequently the pulse charge is zero. The pulse charge is perhaps most important when considering the effects electrical current has on the nonexcitable tissues of the body, such as blood, bone, and cartilage. Pulse charge is related to the width of the pulse in the following way: the wider the pulse width, the greater the pulse charge (Figure 6.14).

Electrodes

Current must be introduced into the body to exert any effect on the tissues. With rare exception, the electrical stimulators used employ some type of surface electrode that is known as a "transcutaneous" electrode. Because it is the interface between the patient and the machine, the electrode represents one of the most important parts of the electrical stimulation apparatus. Many problems that develop with electrical stimulation, including failure to arrive at the desired effect, can be traced to problems with the electrode.

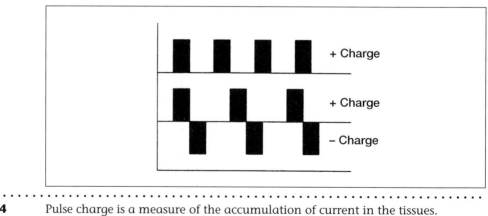

FIGURE 6.14   Pulse charge is a measure of the accumulation of current in the tissues.

Electrode Type

Currently, there are a number of different electrodes that are used in the clinical setting. Each type has certain advantages and disadvantages. Often, the type of electrode used is based more on habit than on any particular rationale. A variety of electrodes that are commonly used include:

Carbon-filled Silicone Electrodes (Rubber). These are probably the most commonly found electrodes. They come in a variety of sizes and are usually black and red (Figure 6.15). These electrodes must have some moist material such as a moistened sponge placed between them and the patient's skin. Some clinicians prefer to use an electrolytic gel or spray on the electrodes. As with other types of electrodes, the rubber electrodes must be held in firm contact with the skin. This is usually accomplished by the use of elastic straps. The advantages of this type of electrode include ease of use, pliability, and availability. Disadvantages include that they tend to get dirty and become less pliable with age, especially when gels or sprays are used as a contact medium. When sponges are used with these electrodes, they should be disinfected between each patient application.

Metal Electrodes Covered by a Moistened Sponge. This type of electrode was commonly used in the past, but less frequently so today. These

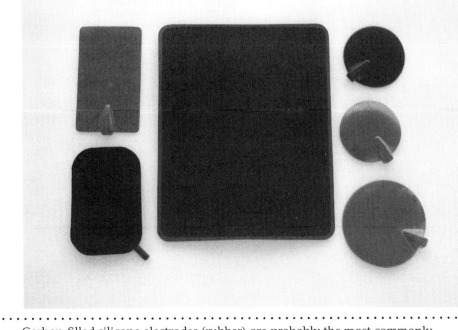

FIGURE 6.15   Carbon-filled silicone electrodes (rubber) are probably the most commonly found electrodes.

electrodes may still be found with electrical stimulators provided by some manufacturers (Figure 6.16). As with rubber electrodes, metal electrodes must be held in place with some type of strap. There are no particular advantages to this type of electrode. Disadvantages are much the same as those for the rubber electrode.

Vacuum Electrodes (Usually Found with Interferential Current). This type of electrode consists of a rubber cup that is designed to be held in place by a vacuum apparatus. Inside the rubber cup is a metal plate that is covered with a moistened sponge (Figure 6.17). The lead connecting the electrode to the stimulator consists of a hollow metal ring. When the vacuum apparatus is turned on, the resulting suction holds the electrode in place. These electrodes were designed to maximize the contact between patient and stimulator and to allow good electrode contact in areas, such as the shoulder, that might otherwise be difficult to accomplish. The primary advantage of these electrodes is the ability to apply them in rough or uneven areas of the body. Disadvantages include the creation of a welt under the electrode and the added expense of the vacuum apparatus.

Self-adhesive Electrodes Made of Karya Gum (Often Used with TENS Units). One of the more recent innovations in the field of electrical stimulation is the self-adhesive electrode (Figure 6.18). Although these electrodes have been available for several years, recent improvements have made them

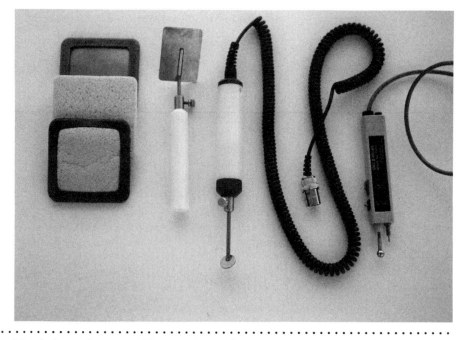

FIGURE 6.16   Metal electrodes covered by a moistened sponge are not commonly available.

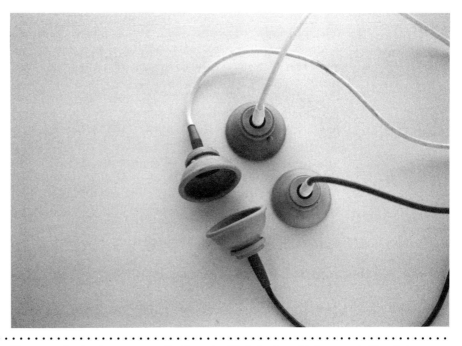

FIGURE 6.17   Vacuum electrodes are usually found with interferential current stimulators.

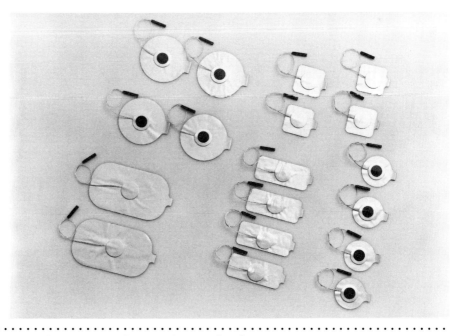

FIGURE 6.18   Self-adhesive electrodes are often used with TENS units.

an essential part of electrical stimulation. The advantages of these electrodes include the extreme ease of use, patient comfort, and ability to use at home with TENS devices. In addition, they are very hygienic when each patient is supplied with his or her own electrodes. Primary disadvantages include the added cost and the fact that they tend to wear out after repeated use.

Small, Metal Probe. This type of electrode is commonly used to treat myofascial trigger points (Figure 6.19). When used in combination with electrical stimulation, the transducer of an ultrasound unit is actually a metal probe-type electrode. The primary advantage of this electrode is the ability to stimulate small areas such as trigger points.

Q-tip Electrodes. The use of the common Q-tip was introduced as an electrode with the introduction of the microcurrent stimulation devices (Figure 6.20). The advantages of this electrode are the ability to stimulate extremely small areas and low cost.

Size

As seen with the various types available, electrodes come in a variety of sizes (Figure 6.21). Size is directly related to the current density beneath the electrode, skin impedance, degree of sensation, and strength of the stimulus in the following ways:

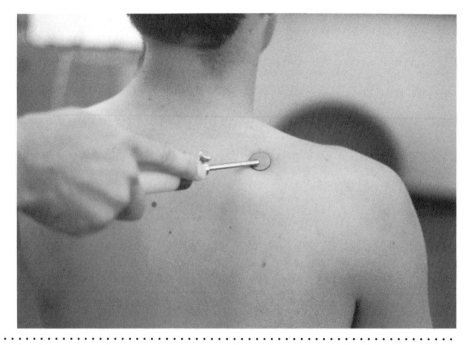

FIGURE 6.19   Small, metal probe electrode is commonly used to treat myofascial trigger points.

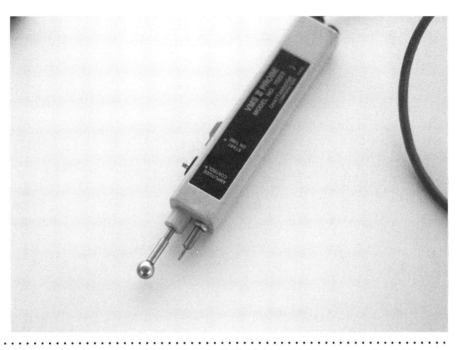

FIGURE 6.20   Common Q-tip is used as an electrode with the microcurrent stimulation devices.

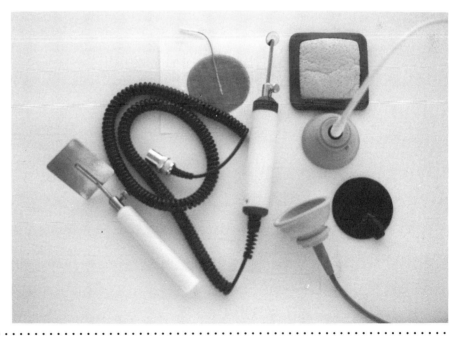

FIGURE 6.21   Electrodes come in a variety of sizes.

- The smaller the electrode, the greater the current density; the current density beneath a probe electrode is much higher than that found below a large 8 × 10 inch dispersive pad.
- The skin impedance beneath a small tip electrode (1 mm²) is between 100 and 1000 ohms, whereas the impedance beneath a 4 × 4 inch electrode (100 cm²) may reach 50,000 to 100,000 ohms.
- The larger the size of the electrode, the less sensation the patient feels beneath the electrode. When an HVG stimulator is used patients feel sensation and muscle contraction under the smaller active electrodes long before they feel any response under the larger dispersive pad.
- For a given intensity, the smaller the electrode the stronger the stimulus. Different sized electrodes can be used with the same lead wires to modify the effect and the comfort of stimulation.
- In essence, larger electrodes produce a stronger motor response without pain, whereas smaller electrodes minimize motor response.
- For acupuncture-type stimulation, small electrodes, such as the metal probe, are used.

Placement

Correct placement of the electrodes is one of the most important aspects of electrical stimulation. If other aspects of the stimulation protocol are set at the appropriate parameters, but the electrodes are improperly applied, in all probability the therapeutic objective will not be attained.

Electrode placement is determined by two factors: (1) the type of stimulator that is being used (AC or DC), and (2) the therapeutic objective.

Stimulator Type

There are three basic techniques of applying electrodes (Figure 6.22):

- monopolar—used with direct current; polarity for each electrode remains the same for the treatment duration.
- bipolar—used with alternating current; the polarity of each electrode is continually changing during the treatment; consequently, at some point each electrode will be both positive and negative.
- quadripolar—used with interferential current; actually is a combination of two bipolar applications that are arranged so that they intersect.

Therapeutic Objective

The basic therapeutic objective, whether it involves a sensory level of stimulation, some form of muscle contraction, or a noxious level of stimulus, determines the location of the electrodes as follows:

Subthreshold Stimulation. When using a subthreshold stimulation procedure for either pain control or to facilitate tissue repair, it is customary to place the electrodes around the injured area. In some instances, Q-tip electrodes may be used over acupuncture points.

Sensory Stimulation. If the objective of the therapy calls for a sensory level stimulus (SLS), such as for pain relief via the pain gate mechanism, the following electrode applications are suggested:

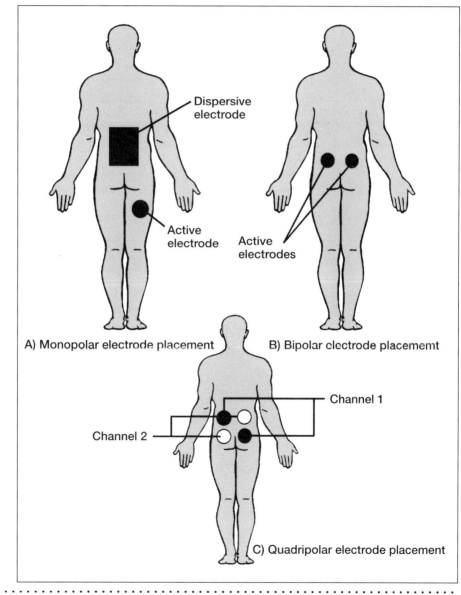

FIGURE 6.22   Basic electrode placement techniques.

- surround the target area with electrodes (Figure 6.23)
- place electrodes at the level of the spine that corresponds to the painful area (Figure 6.24)
- place electrodes along the course of an associated peripheral nerve (Figure 6.25)
- place electrodes along the course of an associated dermatome (Figure 6.26)

Note: When using electrical stimulation for a SLS as described above, both AC and DC units may have similar electrode placements.

Motor Stimulus (Muscle Contraction). If the therapeutic objective calls for a motor level stimulus (MLS) when a muscle contraction is required, the following electrode applications are necessary:

Direct Current. The active electrode should be placed over the motor point of the muscle to be stimulated (Figure 6.27). The dispersive electrode, which is usually somewhat larger, should be placed on a large skin surface such as the lower back or the thigh. It is important to note that when using electrical stimulation to produce contractions of the limb muscles the dispersive pad is best placed in a location that is proximal to the active electrode. The electrodes should NOT be placed in such a manner that current flows through the chest or the abdomen.

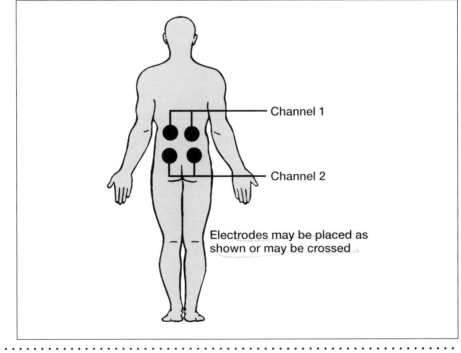

Channel 1

Channel 2

Electrodes may be placed as shown or may be crossed

FIGURE 6.23   Electrodes may be placed to surround the target area.

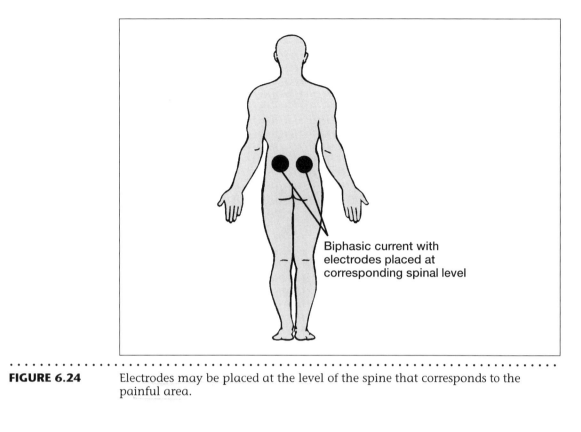

FIGURE 6.24   Electrodes may be placed at the level of the spine that corresponds to the painful area.

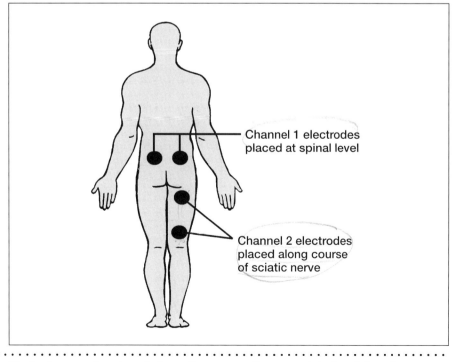

FIGURE 6.25   Electrodes may be placed along the course of an associated peripheral nerve.

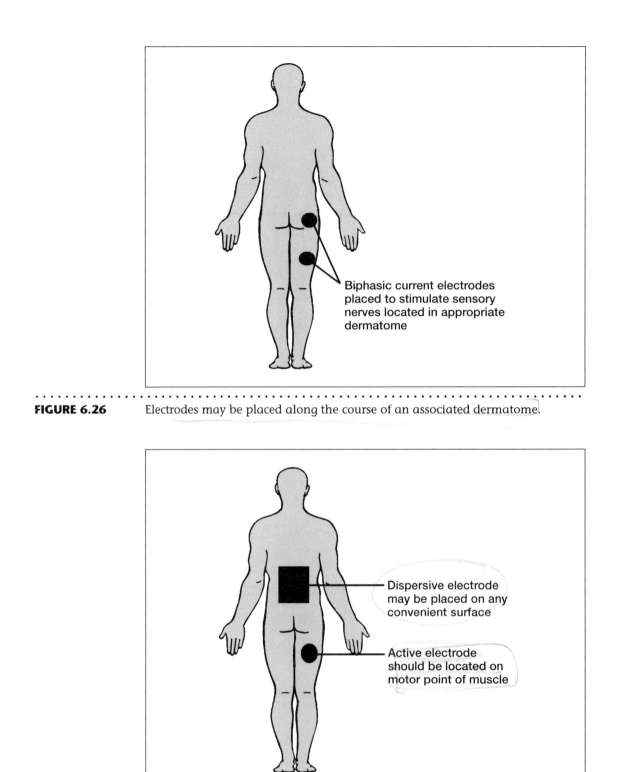

FIGURE 6.26   Electrodes may be placed along the course of an associated dermatome.

FIGURE 6.27   Electrode placement for muscle stimulation with a DC stimulator.

Alternating Current. Because both electrodes are considered to be active, one should be placed on the muscle near its origin and the other on the muscle near its insertion (Figure 6.28). A common mistake involves placing the electrodes on the tendon of the muscle rather than on the muscle itself.

Interferential Current. Interferential current consists of two AC currents that are slightly out of phase with each other. To gain the interferential effect, the electrodes must be arranged so that the currents intersect. To accomplish this the electrodes are arranged in a criss-cross manner (Figure 6.29).

Motor or Noxious Stimulation (Pain Control Technique). If the objective is to achieve pain control using a motor level (MLS) or noxious stimulus (NLS), the following electrode placement techniques may be used:

Acupuncturelike TENS. Electrodes should be placed on selected acupuncture points, which often coincide with myofascial trigger points or motor points (see Appendix B: Acupuncture Points).

Brief-intense TENS. Electrode placement is similar to that seen with classic TENS applications:

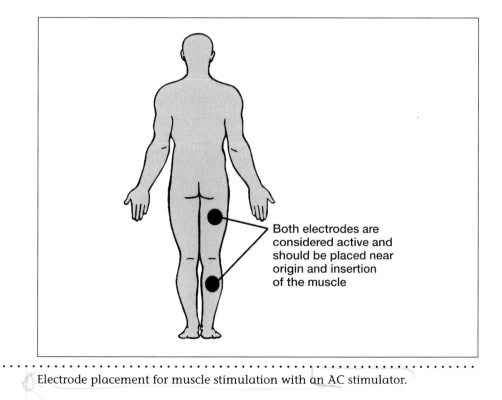

Both electrodes are considered active and should be placed near origin and insertion of the muscle

FIGURE 6.28   Electrode placement for muscle stimulation with an AC stimulator.

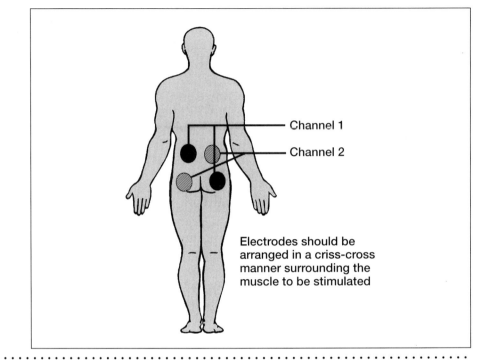

Channel 1
Channel 2

Electrodes should be
arranged in a criss-cross
manner surrounding the
muscle to be stimulated

FIGURE 6.29   Electrode placement for an interferential current stimulation technique.

- surround the target area with electrodes.
- place electrodes at the level of the spine that corresponds to the painful area.
- place electrodes along the course of an associated peripheral nerve.
- place electrodes along the course of an associated dermatome.

Hyperstimulation TENS. Similar to the acupuncturelike TENS, electrodes should be placed on selected acupuncture points. Electrodes may also be placed in such a manner that they surround the painful area.

Note: If attempts to apply an electrical current are unsuccessful, the electrodes and the electrical lead should be examined to ensure that a current is flowing. However, before attempting to test electrodes or lead wires, the current should be turned off to avoid inadvertently shocking the patient. **Do not test** the current while the stimulator is connected to the patient.

Summary

The application of electrical stimulation for therapeutic purposes has grown in popularity during the past several decades. Application techniques are based on our knowledge of the effects of electrical stimulation and on predictable tissue responses. As our understanding of the benefits of electrical stimulation increases, new application techniques and methods may produce a greater variety of uses for electrical stimulating currents.

References and Suggested Reading

Krusen FH. Physical medicine. Philadelphia: WB Saunders, 1941.

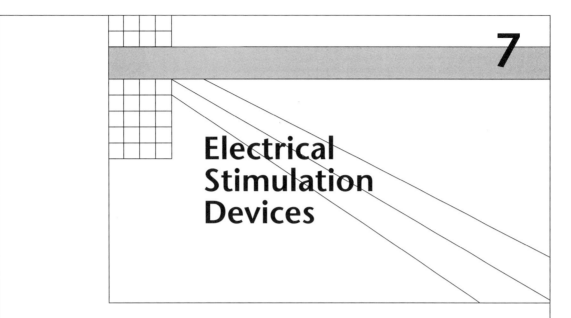

Electrical Stimulation Devices

Learning Objectives

At the completion of this chapter, you should be able to:

1. Describe the various categories of electrical stimulators.
2. Describe the parts of an electrical stimulation device.
3. Describe interferential current based on the following:
   - electrical characteristics
   - unique features
   - application techniques
   - advantages and disadvantages
4. Describe high voltage galvanic current based on the following:
   - electrical characteristics
   - unique features
   - application techniques
   - advantages and disadvantages
5. Define TENS
6. Describe the various forms of TENS.
7. Describe the long-term effect of TENS.
8. Describe the factors that influence the use of TENS.

9. Describe the microcurrent stimulation devices based on the following:
   - electrical characteristics
   - unique features
   - application techniques
   - advantages and disadvantages
10. Describe low voltage galvanic current and the process of iontophoresis.

As the application of electrical stimulation has become more accepted and more popular, the number of electrical stimulation devices on the market has increased significantly. Today, there is a wide variety of electrical stimulators available to the clinician. Each has particular characteristics that make it unique. In addition, each stimulator has its proponents who often support the use of a specific type of machine over other varieties of electrical stimulation devices. Some treatment protocols are type-specific and require the use of a certain type of stimulator. Most, however, may be accomplished with any of the modalities that are currently available.

Regardless of the nature of an electrical stimulation device, the delivery of current from one type to the next has a very similar physiologic effect. Although some of the manufacturers of these devices have participated in research to further our understanding of the role of electricity in patient treatment, others have created problems and misunderstanding with exaggerated claims.

Classification

Electrical stimulation devices can be classified in several ways. One method to classifying an electrical stimulator is based on the type of current that is used (*i.e.*, alternating [AC] or direct [DC]). The amount of voltage that may be produced (*i.e.*, low voltage or high voltage) also is used to distinguish or separate the various electrical modalities. Finally, stimulators can be categorized by referring to some unique aspect of the current that is used (*e.g.*, inteferential current). Stimulators can be classified as follows:

Low Voltage AC Stimulators

- these devices typically use a biphasic (AC) sinusoidal waveform.
- they can deliver a maximum of 150 volts.
- they are one of the more common forms of electrical stimulator.

Interferential Stimulators (Medium Frequency—IFC)

- interferential current stimulators use an alternating current.
- they use two low voltage currents that are designed to intersect and "interfere."
- the high "carrier" frequency found with interferential stimulators overcomes skin resistance and allows the machines to penetrate deeply and provides a relatively comfortable stimulus.

High Voltage Stimulators (HVG)

- the only stimulators that use a high voltage utilize a direct current.
- they can deliver up to 500 volts.
- these stimulators use high voltage and extremely short pulse width, which enables them to overcome skin resistance; they penetrate deeply and provide a relatively comfortable stimulus.

In the past, it has been customary to refer to these stimulators as "high voltage galvanic stimulators"; this inaccurate use of the term "galvanic" has led many therapists to claim a significant polarizing effect for HVG machines. Although these stimulators use a direct current, there is only a minimal polarizing effect and they are not capable of iontophoresis.

TENS (Transcutaneous Electrical Nerve Stimulators)

- the term **TENS** is usually associated with small, patient held, battery-operated units that are used for outpatient pain control.
- TENS units use either AC or DC currents, but all of the small devices that are provided for patients for home care use a direct current, usually run by a 9 volt battery.
- all of the electrical stimulators currently available to the chiropractor are actually TENS units in that they use a "transcutaneous" type of electrode.

Microamperage Stimulation Devices

- these devices use subthreshold current.
- they usually are associated with devices designed to promote tissue healing.
- they are not used to stimulate nerves as do more traditional forms of electrical stimulation.
- they may provide the most promising form of electrical stimulation.

Low Voltage Galvanic (LVG) Stimulation Devices

- they use a low voltage, nonpulsed, direct current.
- therapeutic uses are limited to **iontophoresis** and **electrodiagnosis.**
- because of the particular nature of this type of current, it is potentially the most harmful type of electrical stimulation.
- they are not usually considered a very comfortable form of electrical stimulation.

Parts of Electrical Stimulators

As stated, there is a wide variety of electrical stimulators available. Although each varies somewhat in its outward appearance and in the parts found on the control panel, all electrical stimulators have the same basic parts (Figure 7.1):

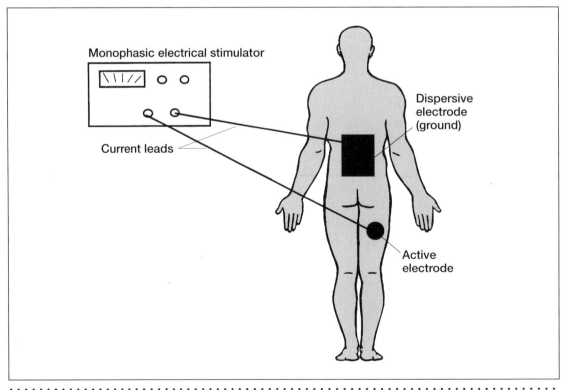

FIGURE 7.1   Schematic diagram of the parts of a typical electrical stimulator.

- an electrical generator that produces the current pulse
- a control panel to modify the pulse parameters
- current channels (from 1 to 4 channels)
- lead wires that connect the generator to the electrodes
- electrodes

Types of Electrical Stimulators

There are a number of different types of electrical stimulators that are commonly used in the chiropractor's office. The manufacturers and advocates of each particular form of electrical stimulator often make claims regarding the superiority of their product versus the "competition." For example, some claim that interferential current stimulators are vastly superior to other types. Others may claim that high voltage stimulators are the most useful. For all practical purposes, however, most of the electrical stimulation devices that are currently in use function by depolarizing sensory or motor nerve fibers. Because depolarization occurs whenever the level of current reaches sufficient strength and duration, it is probably not clinically important which particular electrical device is used. The clinical response is based on current parameters (*i.e.,* frequency, intensity, mode, and so forth) rather than the specifics of the current. The effects on the patient, therefore, are essentially the same, regardless of the type of stimulator used. As will be explained later in this chapter, the low voltage galvanic and microamperage stimulation devices do not function via nerve stimulation. Consequently, the clinical effects seen with these particular forms of electrical stimulation devices are significantly different.

In contrast to the similarity of the physiologic effects provided by the different types of stimulators are the distinct mechanics behind the current delivered. Each of the various types of electrical stimulators has characteristic waveforms, pulse widths, and electrical features that make them somewhat distinct. The flexibility or versatility of individual stimulators may also vary, which may make a particular electrical modality more useful for a certain treatment protocol than another. For example, the probe electrode that is typically found on an HVG stimulator makes it very useful for the treatment of myofascial trigger points. Because most interferential current stimulators do not have a probe electrode, they are not used as frequently for such treatments. In addition, application techniques and electrode placements may vary depending on the specific type of stimulator used. The differences involved in the various stimulators are discussed later in this section. However, it should be pointed out that most treatment protocols are far more dependent on the selection of appropriate parameters than on a particular type of electrical stimulation device.

Note: It is interesting to note that a recent survey showed that the primary reason individuals choose one type of modality over another was their training and familiarity with the equipment rather than any superior effects that could be assigned to a specific form of therapy.

Low Voltage AC Stimulators

Many of the electrical stimulators that are currently used in clinical practice can be classified under the broad heading **low voltage AC stimulators.** These modalities typically use a sinusoidal waveform and are often referred to as "AC sine wave stimulators." The sinusoidal wave has a gradual slope or rise and it is considered to be more comfortable than a square or rectangular wave. Because these stimulation devices use an alternating or biphasic current there is no polarizing effect. These devices vary widely in both cost and complexity. There are no particular advantages or disadvantages for this generic type of electrical stimulation device. An example of an AC sine wave stimulator is shown in Figure 7.2.

Interferential Current (Medium Frequency Stimulators)

In recent years, one of the most popular electrical stimulation devices has been the interferential current stimulator (Figure 7.3). The term **interfer-**

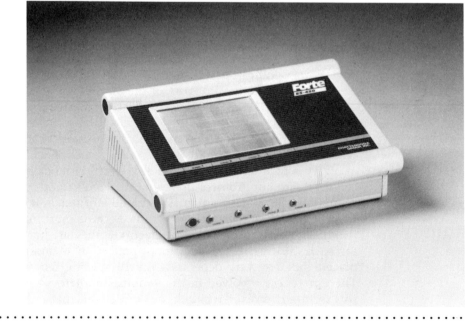

FIGURE 7.2   AC sine wave stimulator.

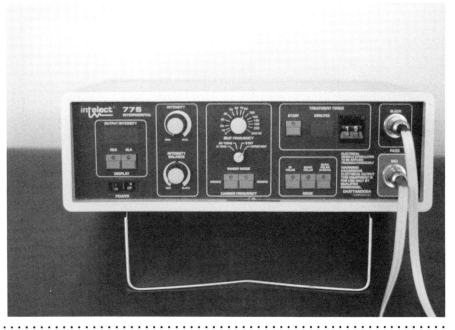

FIGURE 7.3   Interferential current stimulator.

ence current **(IFC)** was first introduced in the early 1950s. Since that time interferential current has become one of the most widely used electrical modalities. The introduction of interferential current was motivated by a desire to produce a comfortable type of stimulation device. It was recognized that skin impedance or resistance is directly related to current frequency. Simply stated, the higher the frequency, the lower the skin resistance. Consequently, a current with a high frequency, such as IFC, produces a minimal amount of skin resistance. This tends to make the application of IFC very comfortable and the current is thus able to penetrate readily to the deeper tissues.

The concept of an interference current involves the use of two medium frequency (1000 to 10,000 Hz) alternating sinusoidal waves that are slightly out of phase with each other. The use of this medium frequency current gives rise to the term "medium frequency" generator, an alternative name for this type of stimulation device. This term refers to the position of this frequency on the electromagnetic spectrum. The medium frequency employed is termed a "carrier frequency" and is used to carry the current past the natural resistance of the skin (Figure 7.4). Most inteferential current stimulators employ a carrier frequency that is in the range of 4000 Hz, although some devices have carrier frequencies that vary from 2000 Hz to as much as 10,000 Hz.

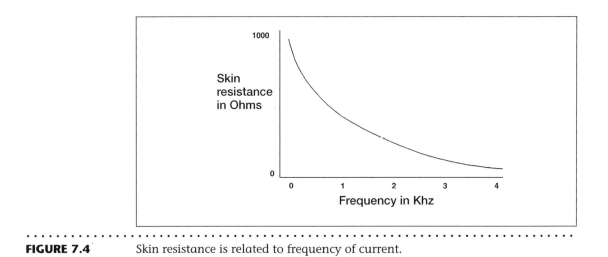

FIGURE 7.4   Skin resistance is related to frequency of current.

Although the use of a medium frequency current has significant value in reducing skin resistance and producing a comfortable form of current, these currents are well past any useful frequency range used to reduce pain or stimulate muscles. Therefore, to create a physiologically useful frequency range that is typically in the order of 1 to 200 Hz, the two currents are modified so that they "beat" together from 1 to 200 times per second. This is accomplished by using different frequencies with each current. When the positive phase of one current occurs at the same instant as the positive phase of the second current, the effect is cumulative and the currents are said to **summate**. The effect of this summation is a beat or pulse of current (Figure 7.5). Conversely, when the positive phase of one current occurs at the same instant as the negative phase of the second current, they cancel each other. The number of times that the two currents peak simultaneously in a second is referred to as the "beat frequency," and the effect on the patient is similar to that of other, more conventional stimulators operating at the same frequency. If a motor level stimulus is used and the two interferential currents beat at a frequency of 10 Hz, they cause the same type of twitching muscle contraction as any other stimulator beating at the same frequency. Interferential current that is set at a sensory level and a high frequency (*i.e.*, 80 to 100 Hz) will have the same effect on the sensory nerves as an HVG stimulator, an AC sine wave stimulator, or a small, battery-operated TENS unit.

One of the unique effects of interferential current is produced as a result of the interaction of the individual, out-of-phase currents. The currents are said to **interfere** with each other, an effect that theoretically enhances the physiologic effect. To create this effect, the electrodes are placed so that the currents intersect and, as a result, interfere with each

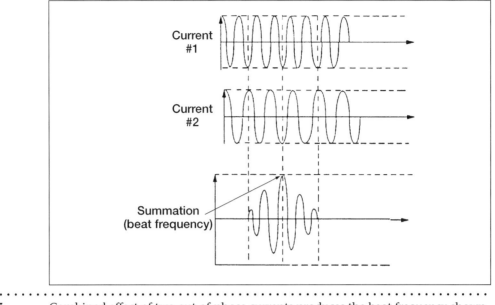

FIGURE 7.5   Combined effect of two out-of-phase currents produces the beat frequency shown.

other. The target area is placed between the intersecting currents as illustrated in Figure 7.6. The greatest stimulation by the two interfering currents occurs in the direction of vectors that bisect lines extending between the electrodes. The resulting pattern of stimulation is said to cover an area that is shaped like a **cloverleaf** as shown in Figure 7.7. By modifying the vectors of the individual currents it is theoretically possible to improve the effectiveness of the stimulation. Perhaps the most important aspect of this is an increase in current density in the tissues. This may be most important in treatment aimed at improving healing times and enhancing tissue repair. It is probably not clinically significant in achieving pain relief or producing muscle contraction.

Static IFC Vectors

One of the modifications used with interferential current stimulators is referred to as the "static mode." With this particular arrangement the intensity of the two currents is gradually raised to the desired level (*e.g.*, a sensory level for pain gate closure). Throughout the duration of the stimulation the currents remain at a steady or static intensity setting. Because the stimulus intensity remains steady, patients usually accommodate rather quickly and this static mode is used when maximal patient comfort is desired.

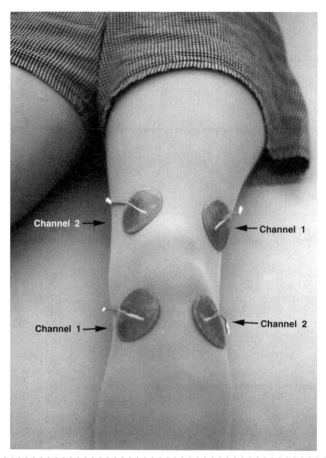

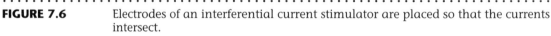

FIGURE 7.6   Electrodes of an interferential current stimulator are placed so that the currents intersect.

Dynamic IFC

In addition to the static mode, most interferential stimulators employ a current modification that is termed "dynamic IFC." This may also be referred to as a "scanning current" or a "rotating field." Dynamic IFC is accomplished by continually altering the intensity of the two currents. After initially raising the intensity in both currents to the desired level, one current is reduced to 75% of the selected intensity. The intensity of the second current continually wavers between 50% and 100% of its original value (Figure 7.8). The effect of this current modulation results from the patient's attention being drawn back and forth between the current that has the highest level of intensity. Because the intensity constantly changes throughout the

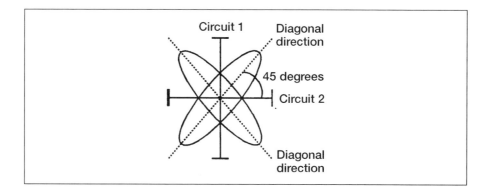

FIGURE 7.7   Interferential current stimulators affect an area similar to that shown by the cloverleaf.

treatment duration, the current appears to move around on the surface of the patient's skin. Patients do not accommodate as rapidly to this type of current as to the static type. Consequently, it may be more useful when accommodation is not desired.

Dynamic current appears to increase the area affected by it. It was originally termed a "distance compensator" and was used when treating large areas of the body, such as the lower back or the thoracic spine. As with most other current modulations, it may exert a greater effect on some patients than others.

Vacuum Electrode Attachment

Many interferential stimulators are combined with a vacuum-style electrode attachment (Figure 7.9). These electrodes were originally designed to facilitate electrode attachment. They were recommended for areas that are other-

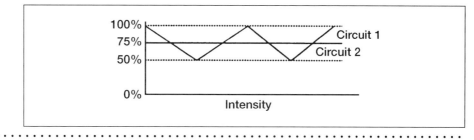

FIGURE 7.8   In scanning mode, intensity of one current fluctuates, whereas that of the second remains steady.

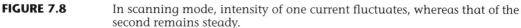

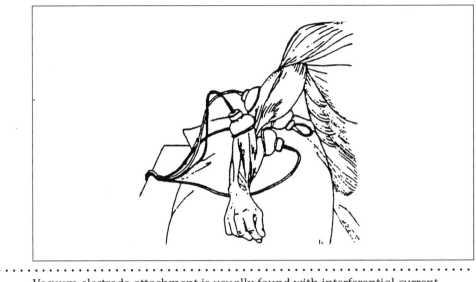

FIGURE 7.9   Vacuum electrode attachment is usually found with interferential current stimulators.

wise difficult to accomplish a good electrode contact, such as the shoulder. In addition to improving electrode contact and attachment, there are some claims that the vacuum provides a gentle massaging effect to the underlying tissues that has a therapeutic benefit. In reality, any such benefit is probably minimal.

Although a vacuum device may enable the clinician to attach electrodes securely to difficult areas, these devices have some disadvantages. Perhaps the most significant of these is that the vacuum creates welts or "hickeys" on the patient's skin. In some patients, particularly those with light skin, these welts may be unsightly and uncomfortable. Although the welts usually recede within a few hours, they may last for several days in some individuals. It is important to inform patients of the likelihood of developing such lesions prior to stimulation.

The added cost of purchasing and maintaining a second machine is another disadvantage of vacuum electrode devices. The vacuum device may cost as much as an electrical stimulation device itself. With the introduction and improvement, in the self-adhesive electrodes, the devices are decreasing in popularity.

Advantages

As stated above, IFC has become an increasingly popular form of electrical stimulator. Proponents claim that it is essential for effective stimulation and that clinical results are inferior when other types of stimulators are used.

Although these claims are difficult to substantiate, there are some distinct advantages to IFC stimulators, including:

- A medium frequency carrier wave significantly reduces skin imped-ance and makes the current very comfortable. Many consider IFC as perhaps the most comfortable of the modern electrical stimulation devices.
- Reduction in skin resistance and the combined effect of the two cur-rents allows greater current penetration to the deeper tissues. In addition, current densities probably are greater with IFC.
- Because of its inherent level of patient comfort and its deep, widely dispersed effect, IFC is best used to reduce pain and muscle spasm, particularly with acute conditions.
- Increased current density may improve the effect of electrical stimu-lation when used to enhance tissue repair and healing.

Disadvantages

Although IFC remains a popular electrical stimulator, it does have some limitation in clinical application, such as:

- Interferential stimulators are designed to be used on a continuous mode only. Consequently, they tend not to be as versatile when it comes to rehabilitation procedures that require an interrupted, surged, or reciprocating mode.
- Some manufacturers have developed stimulators that can be used in an interferential manner and have retained the versatility of other forms of current. Some new interferential units have even been com-bined with ultrasound.
- Interferential current stimulators typically are more expensive than other types of electrical stimulation devices.

High Voltage Generators

High voltage galvanic stimulators (HVG)(more appropriately known as **high voltage pulsed stimulators [HVPS]**) were developed in the mid 1940s, but only became popular in the latter portion of the 1970s (Figure 7.10). Because of the unique characteristics of the electrical pulse, high volt-age devices are considered a separate class of stimulator. Although these stimulators usually are referred to as "high voltage galvanic stimulators," the term **galvanic** is misleading as the current is not truly galvanic. The term galvanic refers to a continuous, nonpulsed current that is used for ion-tophoresis.

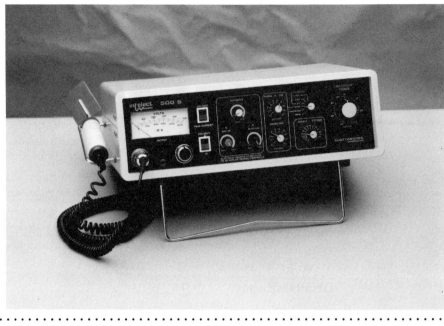

FIGURE 7.10   High voltage stimulator.

HVG stimulators employ a **twin-peaked monophasic** wave that has an extremely short pulse width, usually less than 200 microseconds. Because of the short pulse width, a high peak intensity must be used (Figure 7.11). Many HVG stimulators have a maximal available peak intensity of 2500 mA. These devices combine a narrow pulse width and high peak intensity with high voltage, in excess of 150 volts. HVG machines usually have a maximal capacity of 500 volts.

The primary purpose of providing HVG stimulators with high voltage is to overcome the natural resistance of skin. The greater the force of the electrons (electromotive force [emf]), the more readily they can penetrate the skin. Because little energy is lost passing through the skin, the current density in the deeper tissues is slightly greater. In addition, the extremely short pulse width provides the clinician with an increased ability to select or target specific nerves to be stimulated (discrimination). As stated, currents that use a narrow pulse width tend to be inherently more comfortable. The net effect of HVG is very similar to that of IFC (*i.e.*, it is able to penetrate to the deeper tissues with ease and maximizes patient comfort).

Advantages

As with other forms of electrical stimulation devices, there are several advantages inherent with HVG stimulators:

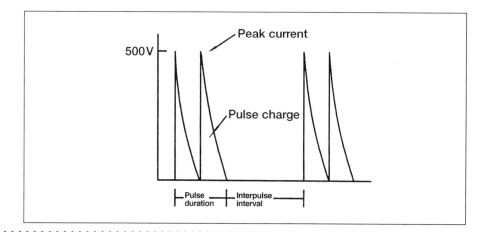

FIGURE 7.11   Twin-peaked current seen with high voltage current stimulators uses high peak intensity and extremely narrow puse width.

- High voltage greatly decreases skin resistance and allows the current to penetrate readily. Consequently, HVG is considered a comfortable form of stimulation.

- The ability to minimize skin resistance results in a current that is better able to penetrate to the deeper tissues.

- The extremely short pulse width increases the ability to discriminate or select between stimulation of sensory, motor, or noxious levels.

- The short pulse width improves patient comfort.

- HVG stimulators tend to be very flexible and incorporate continuous, surged, reciprocating modes.

- Many HVG stimulators have probe electrodes that are readily suited for the treatment of trigger points, and so forth.

- HVG stimulators are often used in combination with ultrasound.

- The polarizing effect, although small, may be beneficial in wound healing and tissue repair.

Disadvantages

These stimulators are quite versatile and there do not appear to be any particular disadvantages. It should be pointed out, however, that these modalities are often employed for their polarizing effect. As stated earlier, due to the extremely short pulse width, this effect is largely insignificant.

Transcutaneous Electrical Nerve Stimulation (TENS)

The term transcutaneous electrical nerve stimulation (TENS) describes the application of electrical current to the body through the skin via surface contact electrodes (transcutaneous). Whereas electrical stimulation has many uses, over the years the term "TENS" has become largely associated with the therapeutic application of electrical current for pain control. The term is often reserved for the small, battery-operated stimulation devices that are used for outpatient pain control (Figure 7.12).

TENS therapy had a major surge in interest in the late 1960s and in the 1970s after the publication of the "gate theory of pain control." With the work of Melzack and Wall, the use of electrical stimulation for pain control became relatively commonplace (Melzack and Wall, 1965). Soon after Melzack and Wall's history-making description of the pain gating mechanism, Shealy showed that direct stimulation of the dorsal column of the spinal cord could inhibit the spread of noxious impulses to higher perception areas (Shealy, 1974). In an effort to determine which patients would respond favorably to such dorsal column stimulation, investigators began evaluating patients with surface electrodes (TENS) prior to implantation and found that TENS seemed to reduce the perception of pain almost as much as dorsal column implantation (Shealy, 1974; Long, 1974). For obvious reasons, surface electrode application is a more widely and acceptable form of therapy than dorsal column implants.

The use of TENS in acute and chronic pain is well established, and a major treatise on current TENS applications was published in 1984 (Mannheimer and Lampe, 1984). It would appear that modern medicine

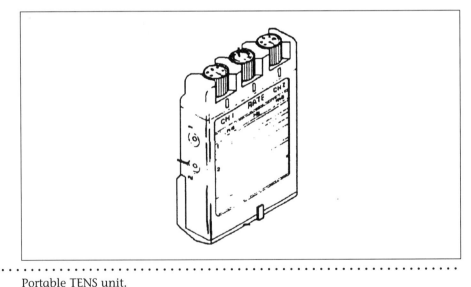

FIGURE 7.12   Portable TENS unit.

has rediscovered a modality that has been in the hands of some practitioners for many years.

It should be noted that all the electrical stimulation devices that currently use a surface electrode are, in fact, TENS units. As previously indicated, however, the term TENS is often assigned to the small, battery-operated devices that are provided to patients on a long-term basis. These small stimulation devices are approximately the size of a pager and are designed to allow patients access to nonchemical forms of pain relief on an "as needed" basis. Most of these devices are designed to be attached to the patient's belt and can be carried with them to work, in the car, or they may be worn while sleeping. They may be particularly helpful to patients following surgery or to patients with chronic conditions associated with pain.

TENS units typically consist of a small device that produces electrical current. Because many TENS units operate on a 9 volt battery, they have a limited amount of current available. In addition, the dynamics of the electrical circuits are not as complex or sophisticated as those seen with more expensive devices such as interferential current stimulators. Most TENS units are two-channel devices that use a square or rectangular type of pulse. Because the available current is limited, TENS units often allow the operator to increase the pulse width to maximize the effect of the stimulation.

Note: One of the current concerns when discussing the use of various treatment modalities is the cost to benefit ratio. It may be important to appreciate that the small, battery-operated TENS units available for outpatient use are inexpensive to produce and to purchase. It is not uncommon to see advertisements for TENS units for less than $100. It has been my experience that patients often are billed excessively for these devices with charges that may be 5 to 10 times the retail price. In some instances, patients have been billed as much as $1000 for a single TENS unit. Such billing practices are detrimental to the use of such procedures and will probably result in challenges from third party payors.

Modifications

There are a number of different modifications or variations that are seen with TENS devices. Each of these approaches uses a slightly different method to control pain and each has advantages and disadvantages. As with any other form of therapy, individual patient response to TENS varies. Clinicians should be willing to attempt a variety of treatment protocols to identify the most effective method for each patient. In the following section we will discuss the more common variations of TENS applications.

HiTENS (Hf-LiTENS)
The term TENS is often associated with the application of a high-frequency, low- intensity current that is directed at closing the pain gate. This is sometimes referred to as **conventional TENS**, **classic TENS**, or **HiTENS**. This par-

ticular form of TENS typically uses a spike or asymmetric rectangular wave with a pulse width of less than 200 microseconds. The frequency range varies between 50 to 150 Hz and the intensity is set at a mild sensory level (gentle tingling). As stated, the mechanism of pain relief is via stimulation of large, superficial sensory fibers (A-beta). The stimulation, which is believed to close the pain gate, usually provides a fairly rapid and comfortable form of pain relief. With this type of application, the onset of pain suppression usually occurs within minutes and lasts for approximately 1 hour after stimulation. Stimulation times vary considerably from patient to patient. They may be as short as 15 minutes in some with no return of pain. Others, such as immediate postsurgical patients, may find it helpful to leave the TENS on for hours at a time.

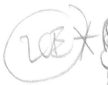

It has been shown that electrode type, quality, and contact affect the level of comfort and the effectiveness of the procedure. Electrode placement is important to effect a positive response. This high frequency form of TENS appears to work best when electrodes surround the injured area or are applied within the same spinal segments as the pain. The electrode position and intensity should be adjusted so that tingling can be felt throughout the area of pain. Electrode placement may need to be altered several times to supply adequate pain relief.

LoTENS (Lf-HiTENS)

This form of TENS is intended to produce analgesia by stimulating the release of endorphins and enkaphalins. It is also referred to as "acupuncture-like TENS" or "noninvasive electroacupuncture." It uses a high-intensity current (MLS to NLS) and a very low frequency (1 to 5 Hz). It appears that the higher the intensity of the stimulation, the greater the physiologic response. Unlike other forms of electrostimulation, LoTENS applications appear to be frequency-dependent with little room for variation. The mechanism of action is via the release of endorphins and enkaphalins and because of the half-life of endorphins, the relief gained is typically longer lasting than that found with conventional TENS. The time required to induce any significant endorphin release is between 20 and 45 minutes. This particular application technique may provide relief in some patients who are resistant to conventional TENS.

Burst TENS (Pulse Train)

Burst TENS consists of clusters of high-frequency pulses or trains (70 to 100 Hz) that are repeated at an acupuncture frequency of 1 to 5 Hz (Figure 7.13). The pulse width and amperage are variable. The intensity is raised to a motor level stimulus (MLS). The strength of the contraction varies from barely perceptible to strong rhythmic pulses. As with LoTENS, the evidence indicates that a stronger stimulation produces better analgesia. The mechanism of pain relief is thought to be mixed with some stimulation of superfi-

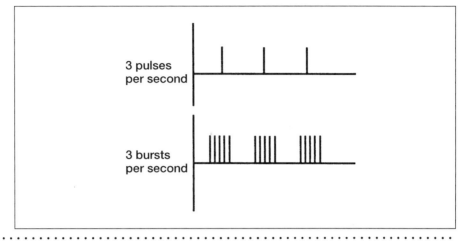

3 pulses
per second

3 bursts
per second

FIGURE 7.13   Burst TENS consists of a series or "trains" of pulses.

cial sensory fibers and some endorphin response. The major advantage of this modification over LoTENS is the level of comfort afforded. Some studies demonstrate that many patients using TENS on a long-term basis choose Burst TENS over most other forms.

Long-Term Effects of TENS

In the early days of TENS it was feared that patients might develop a dependency on the modality. Consequently, a great deal of effort was directed at weaning the patient away from the stimulator. Since its introduction as a pain modality, long-term usage of TENS has received a significant amount of attention.

As with many other treatment modalities, the long-term effectiveness of TENS is to a large extent determined by the manner in which it is originally presented to the patient. The success rate after several months of use varies widely, with some patients receiving significant relief whereas others may hardly be affected. It would appear that the success of TENS on a long-term basis is dependent on the willingness of both the doctor and the patient to experiment with different electrode placements, frequencies, intensities, and forms. As stated, many patients find burst TENS to be most acceptable for long-term use. Some patients using TENS for long periods of time may develop a skin sensitivity due to a reaction to the electrodes. TENS should be discontinued temporarily if this occurs. In some patients modification of electrode placement allows adequate time for the skin to recover. A small percentage of patients may experience skin irritation that prevents continued TENS applications.

Effectiveness of TENS

The application of TENS, particularly in the chronic pain patient, can be enhanced or hindered by a variety of factors. The following factors may interfere with the successful application of TENS:

Medication. Some medications, particularly corticosteroids, narcotics, and diazepam, can deplete the body of the chemicals necessary to control pain.

Prolonged Pain and Stress. Patients who have been in pain for extended periods of time may fail to respond to therapy for many reasons including depression. Because chronic pain usually has a multifactorial basis, it should probably be handled by a team of clinicians rather than a single therapist.

Senility. Senility interferes with patient understanding and the manual dexterity necessary both to connect electrodes and to control the TENS devices.

Patient Understanding. As with any form of treatment, compliance lessens if patients do not understand the purpose of the therapy. Patients who are treated with TENS, especially those who use TENS units on an out-patient basis, should be properly informed regarding the purpose of treatment, the application techniques, electrode placement, and equipment use.

Unwillingness or Lack of Cooperation. Patients who are unwilling to learn how to use the TENS unit properly or who are noncompliant probably will not respond well.

Poor Posture or Body Mechanics. Many patients have pain resulting from sustained postural stresses and/or biomechanical dysfunction. Although it is helpful to provide pain relief for these patients, it is also important to address such problems with appropriate ergonomic modifications and/or mechanical therapies to eliminate or minimize any continued aggravation.

Those factors that may actually enhance the application of TENS include the following:

Wean from Medications. Although the chiropractor is not qualified or licensed to prescribe pharmaceuticals, it is often helpful to modify or remove certain medications the patient may be using. Appropriate communication with medical providers is necessary to determine the most effective pain-relieving approach.

Tryptophan. This naturally occurring sedative, a precursor of serotonin, aids in reducing pain and stress levels. It is found in high quantities in eggs, meat, poultry, and dairy products (corn, rice, and legumes contain low levels).

Stress Reduction. Reducing and eliminating stress helps improve the efficacy of TENS and other forms of treatment. Perhaps one of the most useful stress reduction techniques is relaxation therapy. With practice, some patients may find that they can control their pain without the use of TENS or pharmaceuticals.

Current Modulations. Patients rapidly accommodate or adapt to a steady stimulus. When TENS is used for a prolonged time it may be helpful to modify the application technique by using different forms of TENS or by varying the current parameters.

Variable Electrode Placements. As with varying the parameters of stimulation, it is often helpful to vary the electrode placement, which not only helps to reduce patient accommodation, it also reduces the likelihood of skin irritation.

Patient Willingness to Cooperate and Experiment. Patient motivation is always a major factor in determining response to treatment, whether it includes TENS, manipulation, or exercise.

Improvement in Posture and Body Mechanics. Improving the living and working conditions of the patient may prevent or reduce many of the problems that produce and/or aggravate painful conditions.

Some patients experience a gradual reduction in pain relief with the continued application of TENS. In many of these patients, the effectiveness can be restored by modifying the above-mentioned factors, such as current modulations and electrode placement techniques. In other patients, the application of TENS has a compounding effect: the more frequent and prolonged the exposure, the greater the relief obtained.

Microcurrent Stimulation Devices

According to the Arndt-Schultz Law "weak stimuli increase physiologic activity and very strong stimuli inhibit or abolish activity." Nowhere is this principle more readily applied than in **microamperage stimulation devices** (Figure 7.14). By definition, this type of electrical modality uses an electrical current of less than 1 mA. In other words, the current is measured in the microamperage range.

Unlike the current produced by the classic electrical stimulators, the currents produced by microamperage stimulation devices are insufficient to depolarize the sensory or motor nerves. They are **subthreshold** in nature and patients do not experience either the tingling sensation or muscle contraction seen with other electrical stimulators. The mode of action of these currents, therefore, must be different than that of the more traditional TENS devices. Investigations into the physiologic mechanisms involved has shown that these subthreshold currents produce the following effects:

- changes in cell wall permeability
- increased intracellular concentrations of Ca^{++}
- increased adenosine triphosphate production
- increased protein synthesis
- increased fibroblast activity

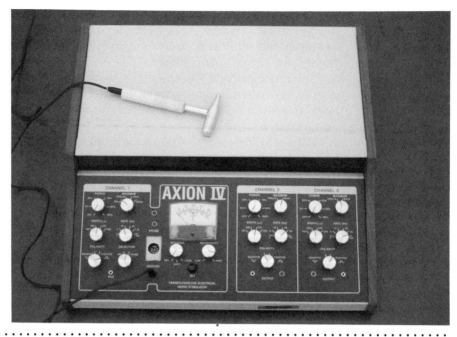

FIGURE 7.14   Microcurrent stimulation device.

Physiologic Effects

Changes in Cell Wall Permeability

Since the introduction of microamperage stimulation devices, many theories have been suggested to explain what has been seen in the clinic. Perhaps the most widely accepted view concerns the effect these small currents have on the cell membrane. It is generally accepted that microamperage currents produce two important effects: (1) "opens" voltage- sensitive ion channels in the cell membrane, and (2) increases the intracellular concentration of Ca^{++} and Na^{++} ions.

Voltage-sensitive Channels. The presence of ionic channels as discrete, ion-selective, molecular pores is well known. These ionic channels are thought to be integral membrane proteins lying in the fluid, lipid bilayer of the membrane and forming an aqueous pore (water-filled tube) lined by polar groups and charged particles (Figure 7.15).

Cell processes require a constant flow of material across the cell membranes (*i.e.*, cell transport). This transport is known to occur in one of three different ways: (1) diffusion of soluble substances across a permeable or semipermeable membrane, (2) diffusion through ionic channels, and (3) active transport mediated by some particular carrier.

Living cells have the property of excitability (*i.e.*, they respond to stim-

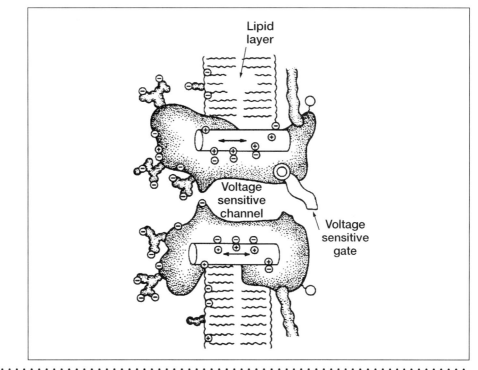

FIGURE 7.15   Voltage-sensitive channels are thought to respond to the low levels of electrical current provided by mircocurrent stimulation devices.

uli in their environment). Excitation involves specific changes in the ionic permeability of the membrane and opens channels, macromolecular pores in the plasma membrane. Channels open and close in response to appropriate stimuli, a process known as **gating**. These physiologic gates open and close in response to changes of the membrane potential induced by electrical stimuli. These channels are termed "voltage gated." The gates in other types of membranes can be triggered by other stimuli such as mechanical or chemical means.

Whatever the precise mechanism, these membrane potential changes must be translated into changes of cytoplasmic free calcium concentrations before they produce an intracellular effect. Thus, electricity is not biologically meaningful except as a regulator of calcium fluxes.

Increased Intracellular Concentrations of Ca++
Current understanding in the area of cell physiology provides the following:

- the cytoplasm of each cell is surrounded by a lipo-protein membrane.
- electric signals are generated across the cell membrane by the open-

ing and closing of ion-selective pores (the ionic channels) in the membrane.

- many cellular functions are regulated by the intracellular free Ca^{++} ion concentrations.

The Ca^{++} ions enter the cell through voltage-dependent calcium channels or are released from intracellular stores into the cytoplasm. The Ca^{++} ions can be called "internal second messengers," as they serve as intracellular links between electrical and chemical excitation and cell responses. Their role is within the cell as a regulator of a broad spectrum of calcium-dependent processes including fertilizing eggs, transmitting chemical synapses, turning on or off certain cell functions, contracting skeletal muscles, and releasing neurotransmitter vesicles.

Increase ATP Production and Protein Synthesis

In a landmark study, Cheng et al (1982) demonstrated that currents from 50 to 1000 µA resulted in remarkably increased concentrations of ATP (three- to fivefold). Currents from 100 to 500 microamperes (µA) yielded similar results. In tissue treated with currents above 1000 µA, however, ATP concentrations leveled off. Currents in excess of 5000 µA (5 mA) were associated with a slight reduction in ATP production.

Cheng states that "electrostimulation seems to increase protein synthesizing activity primarily and independently, although subsequent stimulation of amino acid transport results in an additional increase in the amino acid incorporation into proteins...electrical stimulation directly affects protein metabolism, which even receives an additional impulse from the increased availability of free amino acids." It does appear from Cheng's work that, at least in vitro, these effects only occur during the application of electrical current. A latent effect of current treatment has not been observed.

Increased Fibroblast Activity

It appears that the fibroblast is particularly sensitive to various forms of stimulation, including electrical currents, electromagnetic currents, and pulsed ultrasound. Several studies have shown an increase in fibroblast activity with subsequent changes in production of collagen. Alvarez and colleagues noted increases in the rate of wound epitheliazation, and highly significant increases in collagen synthesis occurring 5 to 7 days after 24 hours of continuous treatment of pig wounds with 50 to 300 µA of DC stimulation (Alvarez et al, 1983). Bourbuignon and co-workers also reported stimulation of fibroblasts in frog tissue culture 2 to 24 hours following the application of DC current (Bourbuignon et al, 1988). Because the fibroblast is one of the primary cells necessary to repair injured tissue, it may represent another mechanism for the effectiveness of electrical currents.

Pain-Relieving Effects of Microamperage Stimulation

Damaged tissue releases a variety of pain-producing substances including arachidonic acid. Arachidonic acid, in turn, is used in the synthesis of prostaglandins and is associated with the production of histamine and bradykinin. Each of these substances can stimulate nociceptors and all are involved in the inflammatory response. Many methods are used to modify this process, including: (1) stimulation of sensory nerves, (2) release of pain-blocking substances such as beta-endorphins, and (3) chemical agents (pharmaceuticals) that interfere with the process. The most permanent approach to relieving pain would be to stimulate the intracellular mechanisms that repair the damaged membranes responsible for the leakage of the pain-producing agents.

Empirically, those using microcurrent stimulation in a clinical setting have become accustomed to its profound pain-relieving properties. It is postulated that microamperage stimulation functions to repair the injured cell membrane which, in turn, leads to a reduction in pain.

Stimulation Parameters

Perhaps the most troubling area in the use of microamperage stimulation devices is the lack of understanding and uniformity of stimulation parameters. To date, selection of appropriate parameters (frequency, intensity, pulse width, duration of treatment, and so forth) is largely based on empirical observations and clinical experience.

It does appear that the following parameters represent reasonable suggestions based on the available data.

Type of Current. Direct current (DC) is preferred due to its polarizing effect.

Polarity. This may be the most crucial factor. It is generally accepted that a positive (+) current is most useful in the early phases of treatment and a negative current (-) in the later phases. This is consistent with the changes associated with the **"current of injury."**

Pulse Width. To make the stimulus sufficient to change the cell membrane potential, it appears that a relatively long pulse width is necessary. Pulse widths vary from 50 microseconds to as long as 0.5 second.

Frequency. Acupuncture point stimulation appears to be most effective at low pulse rates, between 1 and 5 Hz. Pulse rates with microcurrent stimulation devices range from 0.5 per second to several hundred per second. It is suggested that lower pulse rates be used for chronic conditions and higher pulse rates for more acute problems.

Galvanic Current Stimulators

These electrical stimulation devices are significantly different from all other types. The current used is a low-voltage direct current that is nonpulsatile.

Consequently, there is a significant polarizing effect with galvanic current. It is this polarizing effect that is the most important aspect of this type of electrical stimulation. Iontophoresis is the primary use for galvanic current.

Iontophoresis

The application of a continuous, nonpulsed direct current to drive ions (physiologically reactive chemicals) into the skin is termed "iontophoresis." The therapeutic application of iontophoresis is dependent on the polarizing effects of direct current and is not possible to any extent with any pulsatile form of electrical current.

Each electrode of a direct current is a single pole or polarity. The response under each electrode varies according to the **polarity** of the current. The **positive pole** is termed the "anode." The reaction under the anode is said to be similar to that of applying ice. This reaction includes the following:

- attracts acids
- repels alkaloids
- attracts oxygen
- corrodes metals by oxidation
- hardens scar tissue
- decreases nerve irritability
- dehydrates tissue
- produces vasoconstriction
- retards bleeding
- produces ischemia
- provides analgesia
- tends to have a bactericidal effect

The **negative pole** is termed the "cathode." The reaction under the cathode is opposite to that of the anode and is said to be similar to that of applying heat. The cathode:

- attracts alkaloids
- repels acids
- attracts hydrogen
- softens tissues
- increases nerve irritability
- produces vasodilation
- enhances bleeding

- produces hyperemia
- increases pain

Applying direct current for iontophoresis is not without risk; its non-pulsed nature yields a high average current. Consequently, extremely low current intensities are needed to minimize the risk of chemical and electrical burns.

Technique

The application techniques for iontophoresis are slightly different than other electrical stimulation procedures. Two metal electrodes are used to deliver the current and each electrode is covered with a moistened sponge. The sponge used with the active electrode is soaked in an ionic chemical solution. The sponge used for the second electrode is soaked in distilled water. The active electrode is placed in the treatment area and the second electrode is usually placed in a proximal position on the patient.

Due to the strong nature of the nonpulsed current used for iontophoresis, it is important to control the amount that is used. The maximal current intensity is limited to **1 mA per square inch of active electrode** and is always adjusted to patient tolerance. Maximal current should not exceed 5 mA. The **negative** electrode should always be at least two times the size of the **positive** electrode; this reduces current density under the cathode and minimizes irritation. Treatment time should be 10 to 15 minutes for most chemicals and patients should be monitored periodically during treatment for signs of adverse reactions (burns). Because of the analgesic effects of the current, patients may become seriously burned without their being aware.

Note: Patients will not experience the gentle tingling sensation that is found with other electrical stimulation devices. Rather, the sensation with galvanic current is more irritating and may best be described as a "biting or burning sensation."

It should be noted that ion penetration is superficial, usually less than 1 mm. One of the primary advantages of iontophoresis is the lack of systemic side effects that accompany the application methods. This may be particularly important for some patients who may react adversely to oral medication.

Note: It is important to emphasize that the use of iontophoresis involves introducing chemical agents (*i.e.*, materia medica) into the subcutaneous tissues. This may not be acceptable to many chiropractors and may not be allowed in some states.

The types of ions used are determined by the desired physiologic response indicated. Table 7-1 lists common ions and the conditions for which they are indicated.

Precautions

One of the primary precautions when using galvanic current is to avoid burns. Two types of burns may be seen, chemical and electrical. The

TABLE 7.1   Common Ions and Indications

Ions		Indications
-	chlorine	superficial scars and adhesions
+	zinc and copper	skin infections and sinus problems
+	calcium	adhesions and spasticity
+	acetate	bursitis and calcific deposits
+	hyaluronidase	edema
+	hydrocortisone	inflammation
-	iodine	adhesions, scars, and fibrosis
+	magnesium	pain, arthritis, and spasms
-	niacin	spasms and arthritis
-	salicylate	pain
+	xylocaine	pain and inflammation

chemical burns are the result of the formation of sodium hydroxide (NaOH) under the cathode. These may be quite serious and may develop in just a few minutes. The electrical burns are due to uneven heating of the skin beneath the electrode, usually caused by dry or poorly contacting electrodes.

When using galvanic current for the purpose of iontophoresis, patients should be monitored for undue reactions to the chemicals used. For example, individuals with a known allergy to seafood should not be treated with iodine solutions. Those who react to aspirin should avoid using salicylate solutions, and so forth. In addition, patients should be monitored for undue reaction to the electrical current itself. Typically, there will be a mild reddening of the skin under the electrodes that is accompanied by a sensation of warming. It is suggested that patients not be left alone during iontophoresis treatments.

References and Recommended Reading

Alvarez OM, Mertz PM, Smerbeck RV, Eaglstein WH. The healing of superficial skin wounds is stimulated by external electrical current. J Invest Dermatol 1983;81(2):1440-1448.

Bourbuignon LYW, Wenche J, Majercik MH, Bourbuignon GJ. Lymphocyte activation and capping of hormone receptors. J Cell Biochem 1988;31(7):131-150.

Cheng N, Van Hoof H, Bocks E, Hoogmartens MJ, et al. The effects of electric currents on ATP generation, protein synthesis, and membrane transport of rat skin. Clin Orthop 1982;171:264-272.

Long DM. External electrical stimulation as treatment of chronic pain. Minn Med 1974;57:195.

Mannheimer JS, Lampe GN. Clinical transcutaneous electrical nerve stimulation. Philadelphia: F.A. Davis, 1984.

Melzack R, Wall PD. Pain mechanisms: a new theory. Science 1965;150:971-979.

Melzack R. The puzzle of pain. New York: Basic Books, 1973.

Melzack R, Wall PD. The challenge of pain. New York: Basic Books, 1983.

Shealy CN. A new approach to pain. Emergency Medicine 1974;1:6.

Shealy CN. Transcutaneous electroanalgesia. Surg Forum 1973;23:419.

Shealy CN. Six years' experience with electrical stimulation for control of pain. Adv Neurol 1974;4:775.

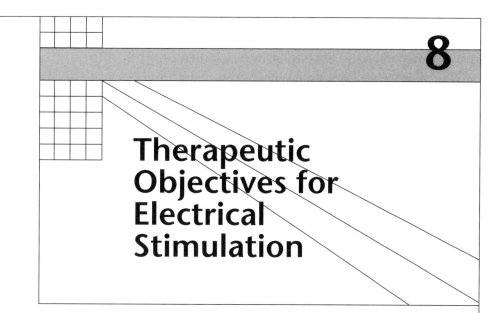

Therapeutic Objectives for Electrical Stimulation

Learning Objectives

At the completion of this chapter, you should be able to:

1. Describe the various therapeutic objectives for electrical stimulation.
2. Provide parameters for the following:
   - subthreshold currents (microcurrents):
     - pain relief
     - tissue healing
   - sensory level stimulation:
     - pain relief
     - tissue healing
   - motor level stimulation:
     - reduction of muscle spasm
     - increase in range of motion
     - increase in muscle strength
     - reduction of edema
     - decrease myofascial trigger points
     - decrease fibrous tissue and adhesions

- tissue healing
- noxious level stimulation:
  - pain relief
3. Describe the treatment process using electrical stimulation.
4. Understand the application of electrical stimulation in various clinical settings.

The application of electrical current is one of the most useful of all the passive forms of physical therapy. This chapter describes specific treatment protocols for some of the more common applications. Although many clinicians use electrical current for only a few selected conditions, such as muscle spasm and pain control, new applications are emerging for this versatile form of therapy. Table 8.1 provides a list of the more common uses of electrical stimulation at each available intensity level.

TABLE 8.1   Therapeutic Objectives for Electrical Stimulation

Subthreshold currents (microcurrents)

- pain relief
- tissue healing

Sensory level stimulation

- pain relief
- tissue healing

Motor level stimulation

- reduction of muscle spasm
- increase range of motion
- increase muscle strength
- reduce edema
- decrease myofascial trigger points
- decrease fibrous tissue and adhesions
- heal tissue

Noxious level stimulation

- pain relief

Pain Relief

Subthreshold Currents

The use of subthreshold currents for the purpose of relieving pain has grown in popularity during recent years. As stated in Chapter 7, it is postulated that pain relief is achieved by stimulating the intracellular mechanisms to repair damaged cell membranes that are responsible for leakage of pain-producing agents. In other words, the microamperage current is thought to resolve the underlying physiologic problems that lead to pain. Whether or not this theory is accurate remains to be seen. However, it is stated that under certain circumstances microamperage stimulation may have a dramatic effect on pain (Figure 8.1). It is also seen that the impact of

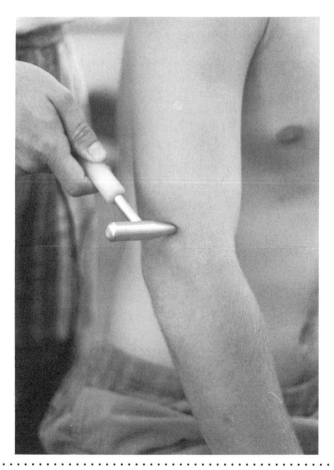

FIGURE 8.1   Microcurrent stimulation is often used for pain control.

microamperage stimulation accumulates with repeated use and it may often take several treatments before any real symptomatic change may be seen.

Treatment Protocol: Microamperage Stimulation

- mechanism of action—repairs cell membrane
- frequency—low frequency 0.5 Hz
- intensity—subthreshold—no perceptible sensation
- electrode placement—surround the injured area, select acupuncture points at the spinal level
- mode—continuous
- polarity—positive for the first few days, then switching to negative
- duration—10 minutes

Case 1: Microcurrent Stimulation

Jim R., a 25-year-old high school gym teacher presents with a history of chronic knee pain. He states that he injured the knee 6 years ago while playing college football. Jim relates that, after the injury, he endured several months of discomfort. He had a series of unsuccessful treatments by a variety of doctors and eventually had surgery to repair a torn anterior cruciate ligament. Although the surgery was successful in stabilizing the knee, he states that he has had a burning pain at the site of the surgical scar ever since. Nothing he has attempted to do has provided any relief from this pain. Evaluation of the knee reveals a raised scar that is dark red and shiny. The scar is sensitive to palpation. Orthopedic assessment of the knee reveals slight stiffness with some loss of flexion. Reflexes and muscle strength are within normal limits. A trial course of microcurrent stimulation is selected in an attempt to reduce the sensitivity of the scar tissue. Treatment consists of three treatments per week for 4 weeks. Stimulation parameters are as follows:

- intensity to subthreshold level
- polarity: negative
- frequency: 1 to 200 Hz sweep
- treatment time: 10 minutes.

Treatment is applied using a Q-tip electrode in a probe applicator. The scar tissue is treated with short applications of current, then the area surrounding the scar is treated in gradually enlarging concentric circles.

Sensory Level Stimulation

One of the most widely utilized forms of electrical stimulation is classic TENS (Figure 8.2). As explained in Chapter 7, this particular variation of

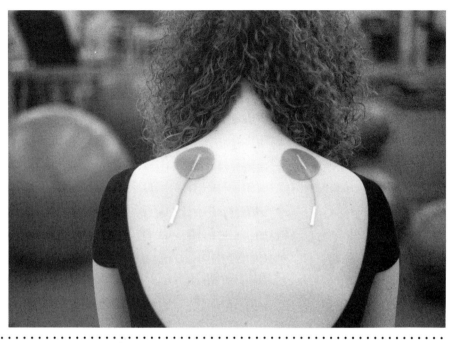

FIGURE 8.2 Classic TENS for pain control.

electrical current is directed at the superficial sensory nerves. According to Melzack and Wall (1983), this sensory stimulation blocks pain by closing the pain gate in the dorsal horn of the spinal cord. Following are descriptions of some of the different TENS applications that can be used to reduce pain.

HiTENS (Hf-LiTENS)

As described in Chapter 7, the term TENS is usually associated with the application of a high frequency, low intensity current that is directed at closing the pain gate (**conventional** or **classic TENS**). The frequency ranges between 50 to 150 Hz and many modern stimulators have a preset frequency range of 80 to 150 Hz. Current intensity is set to a sensory level. This particular application, which represents perhaps the single most common use of electrical stimulation, is used for a wide variety of painful conditions.

Treatment Protocol: Classic TENS

- mechanism of action—closes the pain gate.
- frequency—80 to 150 Hz to close the pain gate (this is referred to as classic or conventional TENS).

- intensity—a sensory level stimulus (SLS) is used; the patient should experience a fine, tingling sensation throughout the painful area.
- electrode placement—surround the painful area, at the level of the spine, or in the associated dermatome.
- mode—either a continuous mode or a surged mode can be used.
- polarity—not usually important and may be adjusted to patient comfort.
- duration—classic TENS (high frequency and low intensity) should produce a desired result within 15 minutes; relief is likely to be short-lived and may stop when the stimulus is removed; longer times (up to several hours) may be used.

Case 2: Classic TENS

Al T., a 40-year-old warehouse foreman, presents complaining of acute lower back pain. Mr. T. states that the back pain began immediately after lifting a heavy box at work. His pain is located on the right side of the lower back at the L4-5 level of the spine. There is some discomfort extending into the right buttocks and the upper portion of the posterior thigh. The pain is graded as a 7 on a 0 to 10 scale and is relieved somewhat when he rests on his back with a pillow under the knees. The patient admits to having several episodes of back pain in the past but none this severe. He has had no prior treatment for back pain and claims that previously the pain has left on its own.

Evaluation reveals extremely limited range of motion with all movements producing pain in the lower back. Attempts to flex the lumbar spine produce an increase in buttocks pain. Straight leg raise test is positive at 10 degrees on the right. Raising the left leg produces some pain in the lower back. Both the back pain and buttocks pain are increased by bearing down. Deep tendon reflexes are normal bilaterally and dermatomal sensitivity appears to be normal. Muscle testing is not possible due to the extent of pain present. Based on the available information, the working diagnosis is acute intervertebral disc syndrome.

Although the treatment course includes gentle mobilization and manipulation, attempts to control pain must take priority. Consequently, it is decided that TENS will be used to provide temporary pain relief. An AC sine wave stimulator is selected and applied as shown in Figure 8.3. The patient responds well to the electrical stimulation and is provided with a small TENS unit for continued pain control at home. He is also instructed on the performance of the press-up as a first aid exercise (Figure 8.4) and is to use ice for 15 minutes every other hour.

Case 3: Classic TENS

Mrs. Molly H., a 40-year-old secretary presents with a history of recurring painful attacks of swollen hemorrhoids. She states that the problem began 10

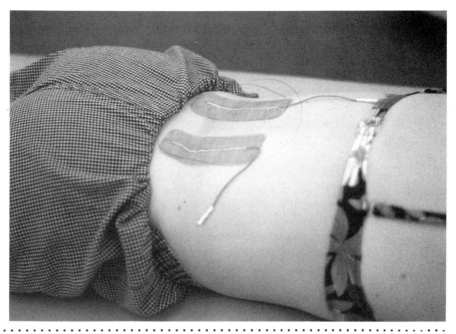

FIGURE 8.3   Use of AC sine wave stimulator for pain control.

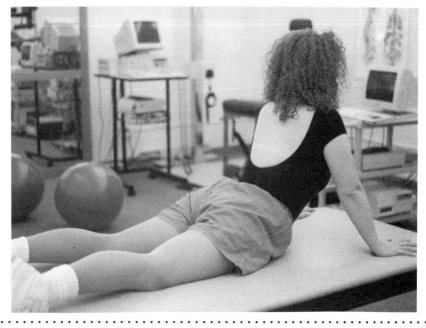

FIGURE 8.4   Press-up may be helpful as first aid for patients with low back pain.

years ago after the delivery of her second child. The problem is getting worse and Mrs. H. estimates that painful episodes occur approximately five times each year. Each attack appears worse than the previous. The pain usually begins during the night and the onset often follows periods of stress or heavy activity. In some instances, she is disabled by the pain for several days at a time. It has been suggested that an operation may be necessary to control the problem, but for a variety of reasons she does not wish to have surgery.

After discussing treatment options with Mrs. H., a therapeutic trial of TENS is suggested. The patient is provided with a small TENS unit that she will use at home. She is provided with a handout describing the application technique and is shown how to use the TENS device. Electrodes are to be placed in a crossed pattern at the lower portion of the lumbar spine and bilaterally in the lower portion of the gluteal muscles. The frequency used is 100 Hz and the intensity should be adjusted to a sensory level. At the first sign of problems, Mrs. H. is told to turn the TENS on and lie down in a supine position with her feet slightly elevated. She is instructed to use the TENS in conjunction with an ice pack and to remain quiet for several hours. The TENS device can remain on for several hours but the ice pack should be removed after 15 minutes (Figure 8.5).

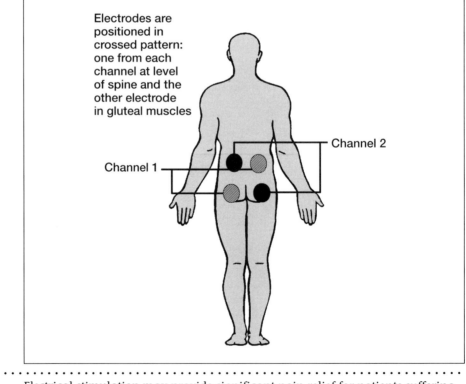

Electrodes are positioned in crossed pattern: one from each channel at level of spine and the other electrode in gluteal muscles

Channel 1

Channel 2

FIGURE 8.5   Electrical stimulation may provide significant pain relief for patients suffering from acute hemorrhoids.

Conduction Block

One mechanism by which electrical stimulation may reduce pain incorporates the use of a high frequency current, typically in the 5000 Hz range. It is thought that stimulation of the sensory nerves with such a current actually produces a conduction block, perhaps the same mechanism produced by pulsed ultrasound and shortwave diathermy. Obviously not all electrical stimulation devices are capable of such a frequency range. This method may only be achieved with an interferential current stimulator (Figure 8.6).

Treatment Protocol: Conduction Block

- mechanism of action—produces a nerve conduction block.
- frequency—5000 Hz to produce a fatigue of the sensory nerve.
- intensity—a sensory level stimulus (SLS) is used; the patient should experience an extremely fine, tingling sensation throughout the painful area.
- electrode placement—surround the painful area with electrodes placed in a classic interferential quadripolar arrangement.

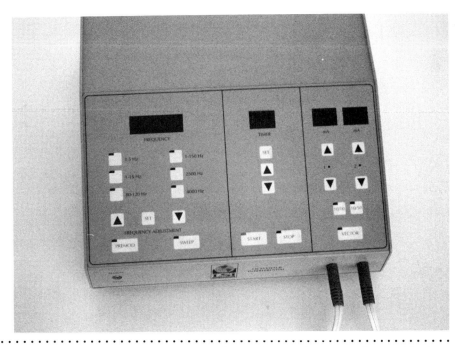

FIGURE 8.6   Interferential current stimulator may be used to produce a conduction block for pain control.

- mode—a continuous mode is used.
- duration—this method should produce the desired result within 15 minutes; relief is likely to be short-lived and may stop when the stimulus is removed.

Case 4: Classic TENS

Jeff B., an 18-year-old high school senior, presents complaining of pain in the right shoulder. He states that the pain is the result of an injury that happened while playing baseball 2 months ago. Jeff is an outfielder on the local high school baseball team and was attempting to throw a ball to home plate from center field. When he released the ball he felt a pop in the shoulder and immediate sharp pain. Jeff was examined by the team trainer and told he had strained the supraspinatus muscle. The pain was treated with ice and rest and the condition gradually improved over the next few days. However, he states that he has had a sore shoulder ever since and he is unable to workout like he should. He has recently noticed that he is beginning to lose strength in the arm. He expresses concern that he may have suffered a more serious injury than was previously thought.

Examination reveals swelling in the anterior portion of the shoulder. It is tender to palpation especially in the area of the supraspinatus tendon. Active and passive elevation of the shoulder is limited because of pain. Resisted muscle testing of both the supraspinatus and deltoid muscles is accompanied by pain. Deep tendon reflexes are normal bilaterally and dermatomal sensation is normal. Diagnosis is chronic supraspinatus tendinitis accompanied by subacromial bursitis.

The treatment plan agreed on involves two stages: (1) to decrease the pain and swelling in the shoulder and (2) to improve the shoulder function. An interferential current stimulator is selected to begin the process of pain control. The initial treatments consists of 15 minute applications of classic TENS with a crossed electrode placement as shown in Figure 8.7. After the period of stimulation, strengthening exercises are initiated within the pain-free range.

Motor Level Stimulus

Although many TENS applications utilize a sensory level stimulus, it is necessary to use a stronger current for certain protocols. For example, the production of a beta-endorphin response requires a strong motor level or noxious level current. Other techniques requiring a strong stimulus level include brief, intense TENS and hyperstimulation analgesia.

LoTENS—(Lf-HiTENS)

The application of this form of TENS is intended to stimulate the release of endorphins and enkaphalins (Figure 8.8). These powerful morphinelike sub-

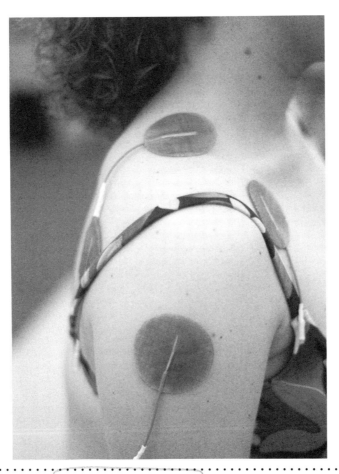

FIGURE 8.7 Use of inferential current stimulator for pain control in the shoulder.

stances may provide relief for patients who fail to respond adequately to the stimulation provided by the more classic form of TENS. Although this particular application technique is designed to use a motor level stimulus intensity, it is apparent that the stronger the stimulus, the greater the response is likely to be. Because the stimulation may not be particularly comfortable, it is not readily accepted by every patient. More gentle forms of electrical stimulation (*e.g.*, classic TENS and conduction block) should be attempted prior to this procedure.

Treatment Protocol: Lo TENS (Acupuncture-like)

- mechanism—induces release of endorphins and enkaphalin.
- frequency—2 to 5 Hz to produce beta-endorphin release (this is often referred to as "acupuncture-like TENS").

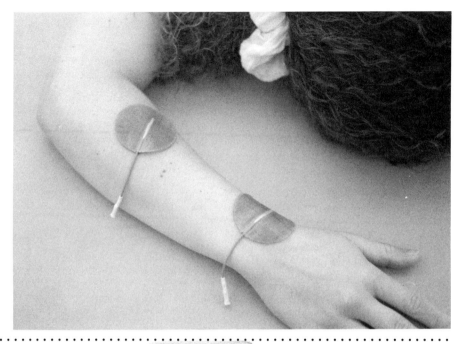

FIGURE 8.8   Electrical stimulation of acupuncture points may be used to produce an endorphin response.

- intensity—a strong motor or noxious level may be used to elicit a beta-endorphin release, but most of the available evidence suggests that the stimulus should produce a significant muscle contraction to be very effective.
- electrode placement—acupuncture points or in the associated myotome.
- mode—either a continuous mode or a surged mode can be used for pain relief.
- polarity—not usually important and may be adjusted to patient comfort.
- duration—LoTENS is reported to take between 20 and 45 minutes to produce any significant pain relief; the relief, once obtained, tends to last longer.

Case 5: Classic/LoTENS

Donna L., a 52-year-old bank teller, presents with a history of chronic sciatic pain. She states that the pain has been present for the past 7 years. The pain began gradually after a serious automobile accident (20 years prior) in which the patient fractured two of the lumbar vertebrae. The fractures were treated with a brace and bed rest. She has had back pain ever since the accident but claims the leg pain developed after a fall that occurred 7 years ago. The pain has been treated with manipulation and various forms of physical therapy, including TENS. She currently takes naproxen and propoxyphene hydrochloride for pain. She expresses concern over the increasing amount of medication that she must take to maintain a functional status. The pain is graded as a 6 or 7 on a 0 to 10 scale. Most days it is 5 or 6. It does not seem to be either improving or worsening.

Examination reveals a slightly overweight woman who moves with some difficulty. Range of motion of the lumbar spine is reduced significantly in all directions. Flexion and right lateral bending produce an increase in the leg pain. Straight leg raising and Faber test are positive for pain on the right side. There is some reduction in muscle strength throughout the lower extremities. There is some loss of sensation in the L5-S1 dermatome and the achilles reflex is sluggish on the right side.

The patient is suffering from chronic sciatica produced by nerve root entrapment. If any significant improvement is to be achieved, the pain must first be controlled. Although previous attempts to treat the pain with TENS have failed, it is decided to use electrical stimulation. The patient is tolerant of the electrical stimulation treatment and the following procedure is initiated: 30 minutes of classic TENS to provide short-term relief, followed by 30 minutes of LoTENS for longer lasting relief. Electrodes are placed on selected acupuncture points as shown in Figure 8.9. After three treatments some relief is noticed and the patient is placed on a series of gentle stretching exercises. In addition, she is placed on a stationary bicycle for 10-minute intervals to increase her overall level of health. Mrs. L. is provided with a portable TENS unit for home care and is instructed on its proper use.

Noxious Level Stimulus

Most patients respond to low intensity levels of TENS. Some patients, however, may not achieve any significant levels of pain relief. Some patients, such as those with chronic, resistant pain, may require aggressive stimulation techniques. Under certain circumstances it may be necessary to use a noxious level stimulus to achieve the desired result. A noxious level current may be used in electrical stimulation of acupuncture points to elicit the endorphin response. This noxious level may also be applied with brief, intense TENS, a form of counterirritant.

Brief, Intense TENS

This form of TENS consists of a brief stimulus at a strong motor level or noxious level. The current is thought to be a counterirritant and probably works by temporarily breaking the pain-spasm-pain cycle. It may be helpful

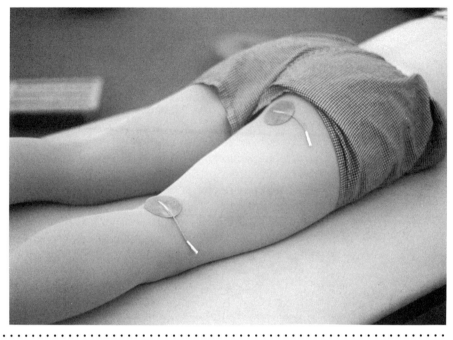

FIGURE 8.9   Electrode placement for the treatment of sciatica.

when other, more comfortable forms of TENS have failed to provide significant relief. It is most helpful in chronic conditions that have resisted treatment. It may also be referred to as "hyperstimulation analgesia."

Treatment Protocol: Brief, Intense TENS

- frequency—70 to 100 Hz to produce a conduction block (this is referred to as "brief, intense TENS").
- intensity—a noxious level must be used to produce a conduction block and the patient should experience a **hot, needlelike sensation.**
- electrode placement—acupuncture points or in the associated myotome.
- mode—either a continuous or a surged mode can be used for pain relief.
- polarity—not usually important and can be adjusted for patient comfort.
- duration—brief, intense TENS is used for 30 to 60 seconds at a time; relief is often dramatic and immediate but, like the classic TENS, tends to be short-lived.

Case 6: Brief, Intense TENS

Allan L., a 35-year-old computer technician, presents complaining of pain in the upper back and shoulders. His primary problem appears to be due to the presence of myofascial trigger points in the upper trapezius and levator scapulae muscles. He is not aware of any particular event that triggered the problem but does notice that long hours at his desk cause an increase in the symptoms. He states that he spends most of the day working on a computer and talking on the telephone. By the end of the day his back and shoulders usually are sore and he often develops a headache. He admits to taking a large amount of aspirin to control the symptoms. He finds that the best relief comes from a weekly massage that he gets at the fitness center where he works out.

Examination reveals a healthy, well-nourished individual with an athletic build. Range of motion of the upper extremities and cervical spine are within normal limits, but forward and lateral flexion of the neck produces some discomfort in the upper trapezius and levator scapulae muscles. Resisted muscle testing reveals some increase in pain in these muscles. Palpation of the upper back and neck reveals the presence of myofascial trigger points in the upper trapezius and levator scapulae muscles. Deep tendon reflexes, dermatomal sensation, and muscle strength are all within normal limits. Diagnosis is chronic myofascial pain syndrome due to prolonged postural stress at work.

The treatment plan incorporates the use of a strong electrical stimulation (strong motor to noxious level at 70 to 100 Hz) followed immediately by vigorous stretching of the affected muscles (Figure 8.10). This procedure is repeated three times and followed by the application of a moist heat pack for 10 minutes. The patient is then taken through a series of stretching exercises that he is to repeat several times during the day. Immediately after the first treatment the patient notices a significant improvement in movement and a decrease in pain. Mr. L is also provided with some assistance in redesigning his work station to reduce the postural stresses.

Note: The following points should be observed.

- for the long-term use of TENS, many patients select a **burst** mode; this consists of a series of a high-frequency current of approximately 70 Hz that is delivered in bursts or packets at a low frequency of 2 to 5 Hz.

- a current modulation can also be selected to increase patient comfort.

- an effective alternative for patients with extensive pain is to combine protocol A (classic TENS) for the first 30 minutes of treatment, and then switch to protocol B (acupuncturelike TENS) for 30 minutes; at this point, the stimulation should be halted and at least 1 hour should pass before repeating the procedure.

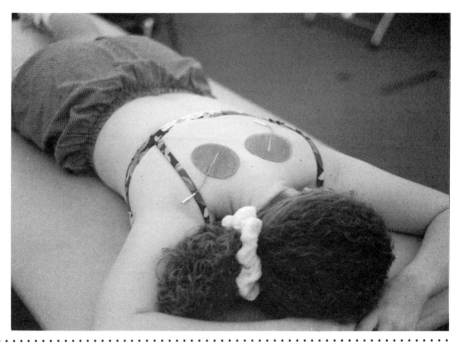

FIGURE 8.10   Brief, intense TENS for pain control (myofascial trigger points).

Reduction of Muscle Spasm

The use of electrical stimulation to reduce muscle spasticity dates as far back as 1871 when Duchenne reported on the effects of electrical activation of antagonist muscles (Levine et al, 1952). This form of electrical stimulation is most often used to treat spastic muscles in patients with deficiencies in the central nervous system. Although this particular type of treatment is uncommon in the chiropractic office, electrical current is often used in an effort to relieve muscle hypertonicity and to relax patients. This may be a primary purpose of therapy or, as is more common in the chiropractic clinic, may be used to make other forms of treatment more effective. For instance, the patient who presents with an acute injury to the lower back may respond best to spinal manipulation. However, the presence of muscle spasms in the lower back may prevent any attempts at manipulation. In this case, electrical stimulation can be used prior to manipulation in an effort to reduce the muscle spasms and make the manipulative procedure more readily accepted.

Electrical stimulation to both reduce muscle spasms and relax tight muscles is, perhaps, the second most common reason for the use of this modality. The mechanism of action is similar to that seen with overuse of a muscle through exercise. After a certain amount of sustained activity, muscles fatigue. The energy reserves necessary to continue the process of depolarization and repolarization of nerve and muscle fibers are depleted and the muscles become incapable of sustaining a contraction.

To illustrate this response, consider the following example; an individual is asked to hold a bucket containing 10 pounds of sand at arms length until he can hold it no longer. After several minutes the bucket gets too heavy and the arm drops. The muscle is temporarily unable to contract any longer and it relaxes. If the individual was asked to lift the bucket and lower it repeatedly, the same response would occur. It should be noted that this response is only temporary and is often associated with considerable muscle soreness following the activity.

A similar response can be seen with the use of electrical stimulation. In order to elicit this relaxation response, the muscle must be contracted with a strong, sustained stimulus. Consequently, a relatively high frequency current (>50 Hz) is used. This is referred to as "fatiguing tetany." The current may either be sustained as when the bucket is held steady, or it may be surged (interrupted) as when the bucket is raised and lowered repeatedly.

Treatment Protocol: Reduction of Muscle Spasm

- frequency—a high frequency (usually 80 to 150 Hz) must be used to produce a fatiguing muscle contraction.
- intensity—a motor level stimulus (MLS) is required.
- electrode placement—on the muscle near its origin and insertion for AC stimulator; for DC, place the active electrode at the motor point of the muscle and the dispersive electrode in a convenient location (not under the chest or abdomen).
- mode—most suggest a continuous application of current is necessary to produce muscle fatigue; some suggest an interrupted or surged current (10 seconds ON and 10 seconds OFF may be adequate).
- polarity—not usually important and should be adjusted to patient comfort.
- duration—variable; the muscle being stimulated should be palpated to determine the point where muscle relaxation has occurred; relaxation typically occurs within 10 to 20 minutes and longer stimulation times may be counterproductive.

Case 7: Reduction of Muscle Spasm

Mary A., a 25-year-old secretary, presents with a primary complaint of lower back pain. Her pain began 2 days ago after lifting a box of stationery at work. She states that the pain is a 6 on a 0 to 10 scale and, when asked to localize the pain, she points to the center of her back. She has developed significant antalgia due to guarding muscle spasms and walks with some

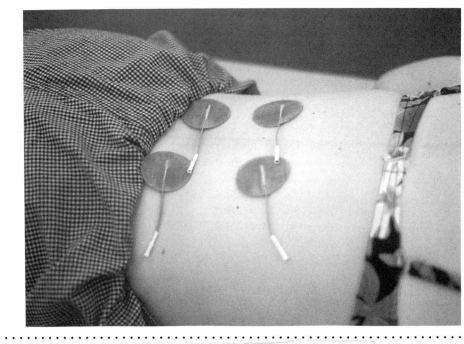

FIGURE 8.11   Electrical stimulation may be used to induce muscle relaxation.

difficulty. She relates no prior history of back pain and states that before the pain developed she was in excellent health.

Examination reveals a loss of range of motion of the lumbar spine in all directions. Orthopedic and neurologic testing is unremarkable. The patient has significant muscle spasms bilaterally in the region of the lumbar spine. Diagnosis is acute lumbar sprain/strain. Treatment will include electrical stimulation to the paraspinal musculature to reduce muscle spasms, followed by manual manipulation of the spine (Figure 8.11). After the manipulation, ice packs will be used 15 minutes every 2 hours at home as follow-up therapy. This procedure should produce significant relief within the first few days.

Increase Range of Motion

Electrical stimulation can be used to increase the range of motion of injured joints in patients who are unable or unwilling to move joints actively. Movement of any limb can occur in one of three ways: (1) actively by direct voluntary muscle contraction, (2) passively by the use of mobilization and stretching techniques that are applied by a therapist, and (3) through the electrical stimulation of muscles. Under certain circumstances, the use of electrical stimulation may be preferred. This is accomplished by stimulating the muscles with a current strong enough to depolarize the motor nerves. The current must be used in a surged or reciprocating manner as described below.

Treatment Protocol: Increase Range of Motion

- frequency—a moderate frequency (usually 20 to 50 Hz) should be used to produce a smooth, nonfatiguing muscle contraction.
- intensity—a motor level stimulus (MLS) is required.
- electrode placement—on the muscle near the origin and insertion for AC stimulator; for DC, place the active electrode at the motor point of the muscle and the dispersive electrode in a convenient location (not under the chest or abdomen).
- mode—an interrupted (surged) current at either a 5-seconds ON and 5-seconds OFF time (a 10-seconds ON and 10-seconds OFF time may be used). (An effective alternative method uses reciprocating [alternating] current with electrodes placed on antagonist muscle groups.)
- polarity—not usually important and should be adjusted to patient comfort.
- duration—variable; the joint that is targeted should be treated for a short period of time, usually 10 to 15 minutes. (Caution should be taken not to overtreat and produce soreness or swelling.)

Case 8: Increase Range of Motion

Gary B., a 35-year-old salesman, presents following an ankle injury. The patient states that he had a serious sprain 4 weeks ago while playing basketball. The ankle was placed in a cast immediately postinjury and the cast was removed 2 days ago. Range of motion is limited due to pain and the development of adhesions. The patient is reluctant to move the ankle actively because of the pain.

Examination reveals reduced range of motion in the ankle with pain on active movement. Reflexes are normal. Muscle strength is somewhat diminished. To begin rehabilitation of the ankle, electrical stimulation is used followed by passive stretching (Figure 8.12). After several treatments, the patient will be placed on a rocker board and provided with active exercises.

Reduce Edema

One of the primary problems that develops in the early stage following an injury is fluid retention in the tissues surrounding the injured part. This may be particularly problematic in a dependent body part such as the ankle. Because fluid is typically moved by a process involving muscle activ-

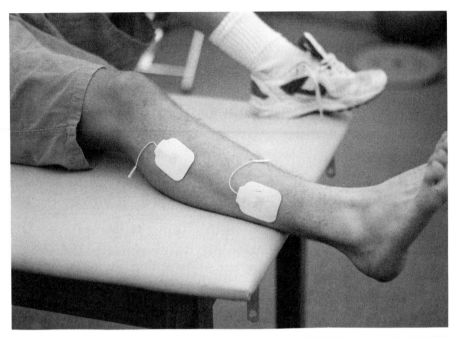

FIGURE 8.12   Electrical stimulation may help increase the range of motion of injured joints in some patients.

ity (*i.e.*, muscle pumping), it may be helpful to use an electrical stimulation device to produce a passive muscle pump. This is accomplished in either of the following ways:

Treatment Protocol A: Reduce Edema

- frequency—a moderate frequency (usually 20 to 50 Hz) must be used to produce a smooth, nonfatiguing muscle contraction.
- intensity—a motor level stimulus (MLS) is required.
- electrode placement—on the muscle near the origin and insertion for AC stimulator; for DC, place the active electrode at the motor point of the muscle and the dispersive electrode in a convenient location (not under the chest or abdomen).
- mode—an interrupted or surged current at a 5-seconds ON and 5-seconds OFF time is preferred (a 10-seconds ON and 10-seconds OFF time is an acceptable alternative); reciprocating mode may also be used.
- polarity—not usually important and should be adjusted to patient comfort.
- duration—variable; typically, treatment times in excess of 10 to 20 minutes may be counterproductive.

Treatment Protocol B: Reduce Edema

- frequency—a frequency in the range of 1 to 15 Hz may be used to produce a twitching muscle contraction.
- intensity—a motor level stimulus (MLS) is required.
- electrode placement—on the muscle near the origin and insertion for AC stimulator; for DC, place the active electrode at the motor point of the muscle and the dispersive electrode in a convenient location (not under the chest or abdomen).
- mode—a continuous current is preferred.
- polarity—not usually important and should be adjusted to patient comfort.
- duration—variable; typically, treatment times in excess of 10 to 20 minutes may be counterproductive.

Case 9: Reduce Edema

Art C., a 28-year-old mechanic, presents with swelling in the left ankle following a recent injury in which the ankle was fractured. The patient was seen in the local hospital emergency room and the ankle was placed in a cast. Mr. C. is able to walk with the assistance of crutches but complains of swelling in the foot and ankle after being on his feet for several hours.

The primary problem encountered during this stage of recovery is the presence of swelling. Due to the nature of the condition and the presence of the cast, it is impossible to use ice to reduce edema. A viable treatment alternative involves the application of electrical stimulation combined with elevation of the leg (Figure 8.13). The electrical stimulator is set up to produce an isometric contraction of the calf muscles. This is accomplished by placing large electrodes on the anterior portion of the calf over the tibialis anterior. A frequency of 40 Hz is used at a motor level intensity and a surged mode (5 seconds ON; 5 seconds OFF). The resulting isometric contraction (or muscle twitching) produced by the electrical stimulation device will produce muscle pumping without harming the injured ankle.

Decrease Fibrous Tissue and Adhesions

Using electrical stimulation in the early stages of injury may help increase joint range of motion and decrease swelling and edema. Electrical stimulation may also be helpful when used to decrease or prevent the development of fibrous tissue and adhesions. Each of these objectives can be achieved physiologically by maintaining movement of injured parts. However, for a variety of reasons including pain, apprehension, and weakness, patients are

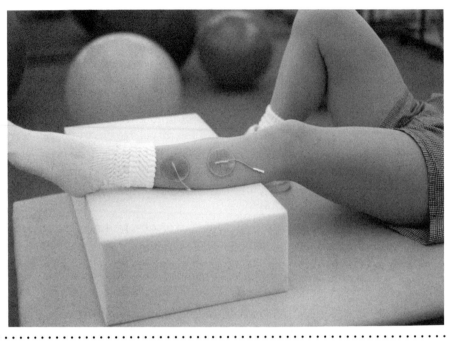

FIGURE 8.13   Electrical stimulation may be used to reduce edema.

not always able or willing to actively work injured tissues. Under such circumstances, it may be helpful to begin the process by using electrical current to passively move muscles and joints.

Each of these objectives requires an intermittent muscle contraction or intermittent contractions of antagonist muscles. Consequently, the protocols for each objective are similar. In fact, when muscles are activated, either actively by the patient or passively by an electrical stimulator, many different effects are produced simultaneously. Electrical stimulation must obviously be strong enough to produce a muscle contraction.

Treatment Protocol: Decrease Fibrous Tissue and Adhesions

- frequency—moderate, 20 to 50 Hz; this produces smooth, nonfatiguing muscle contraction.
- intensity—a motor level stimulus (MLS) is required.
- electrode placement—electrodes should be placed appropriately for muscle stimulation; if a single surged or interrupted current is used, the electrodes from one channel are connected to a single muscle group, and if a reciprocating or alternating current is used, one channel is connected to one muscle group and the second channel to the antagonist muscle group.

- mode—an interrupted current is required, either surged or reciprocating; the ON and OFF times should follow the sequence described in protocols on page 200:
  - acute stage—5 seconds ON; 5 seconds OFF
  - subacute—10 seconds ON; 10 seconds OFF
  - chronic stage—10 seconds ON; 50 seconds OFF

Note: The current should be ramped for comfort using a longer ramp ON in the early phases of treatment and a shorter ramp ON as treatment progresses.

- polarity—not particularly important, and should be adjusted to patient comfort.
- duration—the duration of the treatment is variable and should take into account the stage of the condition; treatment times should be relatively short (10 minutes) in the acute and subacute stages and can be lengthened to 15 or 20 minutes as treatment progresses into the healing phase, or during the treatment of chronic conditions.

Decrease Trigger Points

One of the most helpful applications of electrical stimulation is to reduce myofascial trigger points. Electrical stimulation may be the stimulus necessary to break the pain-spasm-pain cycle that is often associated with trigger points. It may also act as a distractant, much like vapocoolant spray. Once the patient's attention is diverted, the muscle containing the trigger point is more readily stretched.

One of the more useful applications of electrical stimulation is found in combination with ultrasound. Electrical stimulation produces both distraction and analgesia. In addition, muscle stimulation causes a pumping effect that helps bring fresh nutrients to the injured muscle and carry away waste products. Ultrasound warms the muscle and helps bring fluids to the area. Once the muscle has been warmed, flushed, and relaxed by the combination of therapies, it is more effectively stretched. It should be pointed out that the treatment of myofascial trigger points with electrical stimulation or a combination of electrical stimulation and ultrasound must be followed by stretching the muscle containing the trigger points. Without the stretching, passive therapy is probably only effective on a temporary basis.

Treatment Protocol A: Electrical Stimulation

- frequency—high, above 50 Hz
- intensity—a motor level stimulus (MLS)

- mode—a hand-held probe with a manual interrupt switch
- electrode placement—the probe is placed directly over the trigger point; the dispersive pad is placed in a convenient location such as the lower back or under the thigh
- polarity—usually a positive polarity of the probe is most effective
- duration—treatment times between 15 and 60 seconds are suggested; after stimulation, the probe electrode is removed and the muscle is manually stretched; the procedure may be repeated two or three times at a given setting

Treatment Protocol B: Electrical Stimulation Combined with Ultrasound
Electrical Stimulation Parameters Include:

- frequency—a high frequency, 80 to 100 Hz
- intensity—a motor level (MLS) is necessary
- mode—combination
- electrode placement—the active electrode (the ultrasound head) is placed over the trigger point and the dispersive pad is placed in a convenient location, such as the lower back or under the thigh
- polarity—not important
- duration—should be relatively short (5 to 8 minutes) and should be followed with stretching of the affected muscle; there is evidence that shorter treatment times (2 to 3 minutes) may provide adequate stimulation

Ultrasound Parameters Include:

- intensity—settings should be consistent with those presented in the section on therapeutic ultrasound:
  - thin skin such as forearm or ankle, 1.0 to 1.5 w/cm^2
  - thick skin such as the thigh or buttocks, 1.5 to 2.0 w/cm^2
- duty cycle—continuous

Note: When using this combination, the ultrasound head becomes the active electrode. It is important that the usual precautions for ultrasound be followed. The combined effect of deep heat, electrical stimulation, and manual stretching makes this an effective procedure for myofascial trigger points.

Case 10: Decrease Trigger Points

Jane E., a 42-year-old executive, presents complaining of a history of chronic lower back and hip pain. She states that the problem has been present for several years and that it appears to have worsened recently. She does not know what created the pain but feels it may be associated with her running. Ms. E. is a hard working individual who runs both for exercise and to reduce her stress. She is concerned that the pain in her hip may prevent her from accomplishing her goal to run in a marathon. She describes the back pain as an ache and states that her back is stiff in the morning and that it hurts more during cold or wet weather. She rates the back pain as a 3 or 4 on a 0 to 10 scale. The hip pain is more throbbing in nature and is particularly evident after a long run or after long periods of sitting. She states that sometimes the pain radiates down the back of the right leg.

Examination reveals a healthy individual with an athletic build. Range of motion of the lumbar spine is somewhat reduced because of muscle shortening. Full flexion is accompanied by some discomfort in the lower back. Straight leg raising reveals some shortening of the hamstrings bilaterally. Both the Faber and the Thomas test produce pain in the region of the piriformis on the right side. Palpation of the piriformis muscle reveals extreme tenderness and produces some radiation of pain into the right posterior thigh. Diagnosis is chronic piriformis syndrome with lumbalgia.

The treatment plan includes a combination of ultrasound and electrical stimulation directed at the myofascial trigger points in the piriformis muscle. This combination treatment will be combined with a vigorous stretching of the piriformis. The patient will be treated three times weekly for 3 weeks. During the treatment time the patient will be provided with a series of home stretching exercises for the hamstrings, lower back extensor muscles, psoas, and gastroc/soleus muscles.

Muscle Strengthening

Recently, interest in the use of electrical stimulation to improve muscle strength has inceased. Although the therapeutic application of electrical stimulation for muscle strengthening in patients is not uncommon, its use in healthy persons is somewhat controversial. Interest in this area grew during the mid 1970s when reports of training protocols were made public. Since that time, the use of specific protocols and electrical stimulation devices that are designed for muscle strengthening has become widespread. Currently, electrical stimulation has been shown to be nearly as effective as voluntary exercise for strengthening healthy muscle. Some muscle stimulation protocols appear to produce greater strength gains than voluntary exercise. There appears to be no added benefit to combining electrical stimulation with exercise over using either modality alone.

Russian Stimulation

The term **Russian stimulation** has become synonymous with the use of electrical stimulation in combination with exercise for muscle strengthening. This is largely because of the work of Yakov Kots who, in 1977, described significant strength gains resulting from a combination of electrical stimulation and voluntary contraction. At a symposium, Kots (1977, unpublished) claimed to produce intense muscle contractions with no discomfort using electrical stimulation in combination with exercise. Training sessions of 3 to 4 weeks were reported to produce 30% to 40% strength gains as well as functional gains. Endurance was reported to increase after 6 to 8 weeks. Other investigators have been unable to produce the same gains described by Kots, leading some to reject his claims. Kots states that the specific current parameters have not been reproduced, a fact that prevents others from duplicating his work (Kots, personal communication).

Although the parameters of this particular type of current may vary among devices and clinicians, Russian stimulation typically consists of a 2500-Hz alternating current with a burst frequency of 50 to 75 bursts per second (bps) and a 15-seconds to 50 seconds ON and OFF ratio. Electrodes may be placed on primary muscle groups and/or on agonist antagonist groups. It does appear that the intensity of contraction is positively correlated to strength gains. The stronger the contraction, the greater the gain. In addition, there is a relationship between phase charge and the ability to produce torque. Wider pulse widths, which are associated with a greater pulse charge, are more useful. Because both strong muscle contraction and wide pulses are necessary to produce significant strength gains, patient comfort is a limiting factor.

Treatment Protocols: Muscle Strengthening

- frequency—2500 Hz with a burst frequency of 50 to 75 bps
- intensity—a strong motor level (MLS) at the maximal tolerable level is necessary
- mode—surged or reciprocating; 10 to 15 seconds ON and 50 to 120 seconds OFF
- electrode placement—electrodes are placed on the muscles near the origin and insertion
- polarity—not important
- phase duration—20 to 1000 microseconds (the longer the better)
- duration—the duration of stimulus is determined by the number of contractions desired; 10 contractions at maximal tolerable intensity is suggested, repeated three times per week

Case 11: Muscle Strengthening

A 22-year-old man presents complaining of right knee pain. He states that he runs approximately 30 miles per week and the pain has recently interfered with his workouts. The pain began about 2 weeks ago after a particularly long run. The pain is most obvious when he runs down hill, but he has recently noticed some difficulty after sitting for long periods.

Examination reveals a healthy individual with an athletic build. Active range of motion of the knee is normal but there is some discomfort at the extremes of flexion and extension. Hamstring strength appears normal but there is a weakness in the vastus medialis of the quadriceps. Palpation of the knee reveals tenderness when compressing the patella. Diagnosis is chondromalacia patella. It is concluded that the condition is due to a tracking disorder involving weakness of the vastus medialis.

A treatment regimen using Russian stimulation was initiated to strengthen the vastus medialis. Treatment consisted of 10-minute sessions of electrical stimulation three times per week for 6 weeks. No running was allowed during this period. After 3 weeks of electrical stimulation, the patient was encouraged to begin walking, then running again.

Tissue Healing

The process of using electrical stimulation to enhance tissue healing is referred to as "electrical stimulation for tissue repair" (ESTR). In fact, electrical stimulation has been used to promote tissue healing for many years. Although this is one of the less common uses of electrical stimulation, interest in it has grown during recent years. Electrical current is now used to stimulate bone growth in fracture sites that are prone to nonunion. It is also used to reduce decubitus ulcers and to promote wound healing.

Electrical stimulation is thought to improve tissue healing by improving microcirculation. This may occur either reflexively by activating autonomic nerves, and/or by producing a muscle pumping action. Electrical current can also augment the naturally occurring **current of injury**, a relative negativity of injured tissue existing in intact areas (Becker, Shelden 1985).

The methods of electrical stimulation most commonly used to promote bone growth are (1) placement of cathode in the fracture site with a transcutaneous anode, (2) implantation of both cathode and anode, and (3) the use of pulsed electromagnetic fields (PEMF). This last type uses induction coils similar to those used by the shortwave diathermy apparatus. Recently, transcutaneous bone growth stimulators have been introduced that use sinusoidal AC currents, pulsed currents, and interferential currents.

Treatment Protocol A: Tissue Healing
It has been shown that the following parameters can be effective:

- frequency—wide sweep from 1 to 200 Hz
- intensity—either a sensory level (SLS) or a motor level (MLS)
- mode—surged or continuous
- polarity—both poles have been shown to be effective, depending on the condition to be treated

Treatment Protocol B: Tissue Healing

- frequency—0.1 to 20 Hz for 15 to 20 minutes followed by 20 to 150 Hz for 15 to 20 minutes
- intensity—a mild sensory level (SLS)
- mode—continuous
- electrode placement—quadripolar over the area to be affected

Case 12: Tissue Healing

A 65-year-old patient presents with a surgical scar that has not healed well. The scar is the result of an operation 3 months ago for an inguinal hernia. The scar is red and swollen and painful to the touch. The patient states that he has used a variety of salves and medications to reduce the swelling, but so far nothing appears to help. It is decided to use a series of electrical stimulation treatments to attempt to facilitate the healing of the surgical scar. An interferential current stimulator is selected and electrodes are placed in a crossed manner surrounding the scar. A wide frequency sweep (1 to 200 Hz) is used at a mild sensory level. Treatment is scheduled three times per week for 4 weeks. Each treatment is 20 minutes.

Summary

Electrical stimulation remains one of the most useful and versatile forms of physical therapy (Table 8.2). As with other modalities, successful treatment procedures are dependent on a number of factors including the accuracy of the diagnosis, the clinician's skill and confidence, and patient motivation. It is important to emphasize that, although electrical stimulation is an effective and versatile therapeutic tool, it is rarely the only solution. Often, by eliminating or improving symptoms, the electrical stimulation procedure provides an opportunity for the chiropractor to address the underlying causes of the problem.

TABLE 8.2   Treatment Procedure

Step 1:	Determine the therapeutic objective
Step 2:	Position the patient in a comfortable manner (this may be extremely important for lengthy treatments)
Step 3:	Place the electrodes in an appropriate location
Step 4:	Turn on the power to the machine (although most machines have built-in safety features that prevent shocking the patient, it is a good idea to develop the habit of turning all of the dials back to zero prior to turning the machine on)
Step 5:	Set the appropriate parameters: frequency, mode, polarity, duration
Step 6:	Start the current flow
Step 7:	Raise the intensity to the desired physiologic response (SLS, MLS, NLS), which should always be accompanied by the statement "to patient tolerance."

References and Suggested Reading

Becker RO, Shelden G. The body electric: electromagnetism and the foundation of life. New York: Wm. Morrow, 1985.

Levine MG, Knott M, Kabot H. Relaxation of spasticity by electrical stimulation of antagonist muscles. Arch Phys Med 1952;33:668-673.

Melzock R, Wall PD. The challenge of pain. New York: Basic Books, 1983.

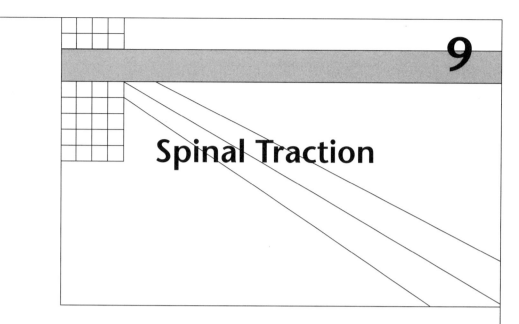

Spinal Traction

Learning Objectives

At the completion of this chapter, you should be able to:

1. Define traction.
2. Describe the physiologic effects of spinal traction.
3. Describe the various types of spinal traction including:
   - continuous traction
   - sustained (static) traction
   - intermittent traction
   - manual traction
   - positional traction
   - autotraction
   - gravity lumbar traction
   - flexion-distraction technique
   - intersegmental traction
4. Describe the indications and contraindications for spinal traction.
5. Describe the precautions when using spinal traction.
6. Describe the traction techniques for the lumbar spine using the following:

- patient position
- angle of pull
- duration
- frequency of treatment

7. Describe the traction techniques for the cervical spine using the following:

- patient position
- angle of pull
- duration
- frequency of treatment

8. Describe the techniques for using cervical over-the-door traction.

Traction is defined as "the act of drawing." As a form of therapy, it involves the application of both manual and mechanical forces to draw adjacent body parts away from each other. The resulting separation can decompress irritated tissues, realign parts, and relax tight structures. Traction is one of the oldest methods of therapy known and has been employed in a variety of forms since ancient times. Early civilizations used a variety of traction devices in an effort to relieve pain and discomfort (Figure 9.1). Many of these early forms of traction may seem barbaric, even cruel, yet traction has remained a common form of therapy for many conditions, particularly low back pain. In more recent times, the therapeutic application of traction has been enhanced by improvements in both equipment and protocols.

Currently, traction is used for a variety of disorders. In medicine, it is perhaps most frequently used in the treatment of fractures and dislocations. For the chiropractor, traction in all of its various forms is most often used in the treatment of spinal disorders such as intervertebral disc herniations.

Effects of Spinal Traction

Although some forms of traction are applied to the bones and joints of the extremities (*e.g.*, fractures), in this section we focus on the application of traction to the spine. Correctly performed, traction can cause any or all of the following effects:

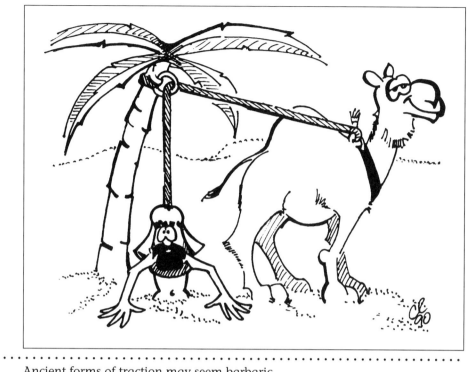

FIGURE 9.1   Ancient forms of traction may seem barbaric.

- distraction or separation of the vertebral bodies
- a combined action of distraction and gliding of facet articulations
- tensing of the ligaments of the spine
- widening of the intervertebral foramen
- straightening of spinal curves
- stretching of spinal musculature

Types of Spinal Traction

There are a variety of traction devices and procedures used in a chiropractor's office. Some of these procedures are fairly common (*e.g.*, manual traction) whereas others are used less frequently (*e.g.*, inversion therapy). As with other forms of therapy, each of the various forms of traction has specific applications and may elicit a positive effect on selected conditions. Each form of traction has advantages and disadvantages and one that is appropriate for one patient may not be so for another.

Continuous Traction

This particular form of traction involves light weight applied for prolonged periods of time. It is generally accepted that this form is ineffective at producing separation because of the slight force used. Continuous traction is generally used to align and stabilize adjacent body parts when there are fractures and/or dislocations. It is used primarily in the spine for cervical fractures and is not typically applied by chiropractors.

An example of continuous spinal traction is the halo type device used following a fracture of the cervical spine. It may also be used after certain surgical procedures such as spinal fusions. With this particular method, small holes are drilled into the skull. These holes are used to attach the traction device to the head of the patient. The remainder of the device is firmly attached to the upper trunk with a harness. The objectives of the device are to stabilize the cervical spine, to maintain alignment of the cervical structures during healing, and to prevent movement between adjacent structures.

Sustained (Static) Traction

As with continuous traction, sustained traction applies a constant amount of force. In contrast, however, sustained traction is used for a much shorter period of time—from only a few minutes to as long as 30 minutes. The shorter duration seen with static traction is coupled with a greater traction force than that seen with continuous traction. Static traction is used mostly for intervertebral disc herniations and may be effectively applied in both the cervical and lumbar spine. Sustained traction is probably most helpful in the early phases of treatment when there is significant guarding and muscle spasm present. As the patient's condition improves, intermittent traction may prove to be more helpful. (Specific application techniques for sustained traction will be described later in this chapter.)

In addition to the traction devices used in the chiropractic clinic, the home cervical traction units (over-door) are examples of sustained traction. These devices use a traction force that ranges from 5 to 15 pounds. Although the forces probably are not great enough to create any significant separation, many patients find these devices helpful. (The over-door traction device will be discussed later in this chapter.)

Intermittent Traction

One common modification of spinal traction involves the application of different traction forces that are alternately applied and released (hold/ rest). In this form of traction a moderate force is applied for a period of time, usually from 30 to 60 seconds. This is referred to as the **"hold time."** This moderate force is then reduced to a lesser traction force that is applied for a shorter period— from 10 to 20 seconds—the **rest period**. The traction device alternates between the two different forces for the treatment duration, thereby producing not only traction and separation, but some degree of movement. This is probably the most common type of mechanical traction in current use in the chiropractor's office. It is most often used for joint dysfunction and degenerative disc disease. As stated, it can also be used for disc protrusions with longer hold/rest periods (60 seconds hold/20 seconds rest).

Manual Traction

As its name implies, manual traction involves the application of manual forces to the joints of the body. The traction forces usually are applied for a few seconds at a time and, typically, in a rhythmic nature. Although manual traction may often be beneficial by itself, it is often employed prior to other mechanical forms of traction in order to assess the patient's tolerance. Patients who may be intolerant of manual traction probably will not respond well to more aggressive forms of traction.

One effective method of applying manual traction consists of wrapping a rolled up towel around the patient's neck as shown in Figure 9.2. Tension is gradually and gently applied by the chiropractor. After holding the tension for several seconds, it is gradually released. The procedure may be repeated several times and may often provide significant relief for patients

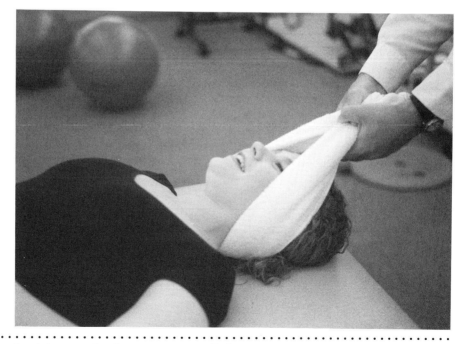

FIGURE 9.2   Applying traction by wrapping a rolled up towel around the patient's neck (manual traction).

with cervical stiffness, disc problems, headaches, and other conditions. In addition to any relief that might be provided with this procedure, it is useful to determine whether a patient might respond to other forms of traction. As tension is applied, the patient's response to traction is observed. Those patients who respond favorably may be safely and effectively treated with other mechanical traction devices.

Unlike most other forms of traction that are used in the chiropractor's office, manual traction is often applied to the peripheral joints, such as the hip, knee, or shoulder. Manual traction directed at the nonspinal joints may play a significant role in improving joint mobility, reducing pain and muscle spasm, and improving circulation. In addition, manual traction may be directed at a subluxated or dislocated joint. For example, the athlete who presents with a dislocation of one of the interphalangeal joints of the hand or the glenohumeral joint may respond appropriately to manual traction and realignment.

Positional Traction

A fairly common form of traction involves the application of variations in body positions, pillows, blocks, or sandbags over an extended period of time to effect a longitudinal pull on spinal structures. These techniques are incorporated into many of the procedures used by McKenzie in his extension protocols for low back pain patients (McKenzie, 1981). In addition, the blocks used in the **sacro-occipital technique (SOT)** are examples of positional traction. A common form of positional traction that is used by many chiropractors is the contoured cervical pillow (Figure 9.3). These pillows are designed to support the head and neck in such a way that they provide a gentle separation of the cervical vertebrae, thereby producing some mild traction on the neck. Devices such as the cervical pillow are often recommended for patients suffering from headaches, neck pain, and upper extremity disorders.

Autotraction

This rather unique form of traction involves the use of a special traction bench composed of two sections that can be individually angulated and rotated (Natchev, 1984). As the name implies, the patient applies traction by pulling with his or her own arms. The patient can alter the direction of the traction as the treatment progresses. The primary advantages of this particular traction procedure are related to the degree of patient control and participation. Disadvantages include the need for expensive equipment.

Gravity Lumbar Traction

Gravity reduction lumbar traction is, perhaps, one of the oldest and most frequently used forms of traction. It employs the use of gravity and the

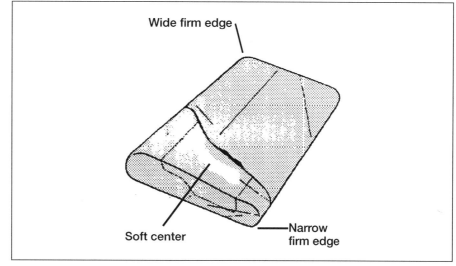

FIGURE 9.3   A contoured cervical pillow is commonly used for positional traction.

patient's own body weight to exert a traction effect. These procedures were relatively popular during the past several decades; however, their application has decreased in recent years.

One method of applying gravity reduction lumbar traction involves securing the trunk to the top of the table. The table is tilted into a vertical position. The free weight of the legs and hips (about 40% of total body weight) exerts a traction force on the lumbar spine. A second method involves inversion of the patient on some type of specially made apparatus. This method was popular for a time as a home remedy (gravity boots). Other inversion devices include the use of the Orthopod (Figure 9.4) and the rack (Fig. 9.5).

Flexion-Distraction Technique

This popular chiropractic technique is actually a mix of manual and mechanical forces. The clinician combines the gentle traction forces with rhythmic oscillations (grade 1 mobilization). These procedures incorporate the use of a specialized traction table that allows the doctor to manually apply and release the traction (distraction) force (Figure 9.6). The **Cox flexion-distraction technique** is an example of this method (Cox, 1992). As the name indicates, the traction force is typically applied with the patient in a flexed position, although some side-bending (lateral flexion) is also used frequently. As with other forms of mobilization procedures, this technique is often best used in the early phases of care. As the patient improves, higher grades of mobilization may be added to the treatment protocol. Ultimately, manipulation may be applied.

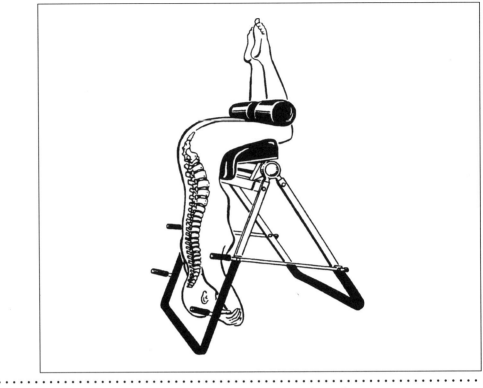

FIGURE 9.4   Inversion traction using a device, such as the Orthopod.

Intersegmental Traction

Intersegmental traction involves the application of mechanical rollers that move up and down vertically as they track longitudinally along the paraspinal structures. The tension, speed, and amount of travel of the rollers are modified to patient comfort. As they move, the rollers lift and separate the vertebral units and exert a mild tractioning effect (Figure 9.7). Although there is some separating effect that is produced by the movement of the rollers, this type of "traction" is more appropriately termed a form of **passive mobility** rather than traction. In addition to the application of the mechanical forces, many of the intersegmental traction tables simultaneously incorporate the use of vibration and heat with the mobilization.

The primary benefit of intersegmental traction is seen in patients who are stiff, tight, and generally tense. This is a very general form of therapy that affects whole segments of the spine. In addition to any mild effect that this procedure may have on the movement of the spine, it is a very relaxing procedure. It is one of the more comfortable types of therapy and meets with high patient acceptance; consequently, it is overused in many practice situations. As with all other forms of therapy, intersegmental traction

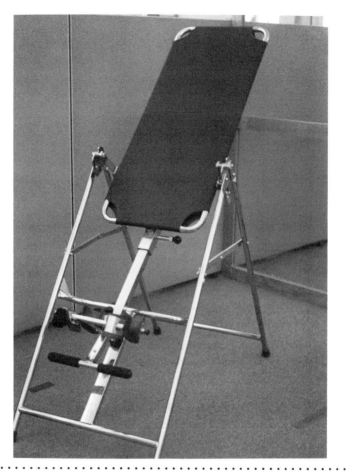

FIGURE 9.5   Traction rack is a recent innovation in inversion therapy.

should be provided to those patients who will benefit from the procedure. It should not be a routine part of the treatment of every patient.

Indications for Spinal Traction

Herniated Nucleus Pulposus (Intervertebral Disc [IVD] Rupture)

Spinal traction is often one of the more valuable forms of therapy used for patients with a herniated nucleus pulposus. Although there is some discrepancy in the literature regarding the best patient position, the amount of pounds to use, and even the best type of traction, the doctor who is willing to experiment with various procedures will find traction a most useful tool.

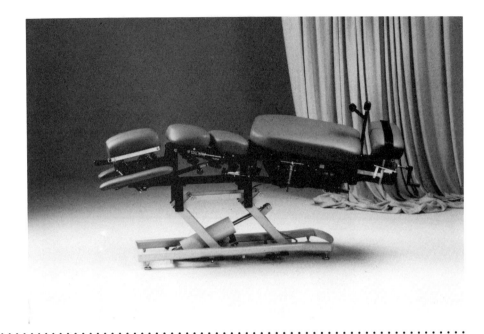

FIGURE 9.6   Cox flexion-distraction method.

There is some evidence that disc protrusion can be reduced and spinal nerve root compression symptoms relieved by spinal traction. A flattening of disc protrusions following sustained traction forces of 120 pounds for 20 minutes has been demonstrated (Mathews, 1968). It has been shown that traction can separate lumbar vertebrae and lead to decreased pressure at the disc space with a resulting suction force (Gupta and Ramarao, 1978). It should be realized, however, that any anatomic correction produced is probably unstable and only temporary. Traction alone, therefore, is likely to be unsuccessful in treating patients with intervertebral disc problems.

It is suggested that static or sustained traction be employed in the case of a herniated nucleus pulposus, particularly in the acute stages. Intermittent traction can be incorporated as the condition improves. Intersegmental traction should be avoided in the patient with a disc herniation until the condition has stabilized and nerve root signs are absent.

Degenerative Disc or Joint Disease

Many patients with signs of degenerative changes in the spine, involving both the intervertebral disc (IVD) and the facet articulations, will benefit from spinal traction techniques. The traction exerts a separating effect that, although mild and temporary, may often yield significant clinical improvement.

Traction produces separation and widening of the intervertebral fora-

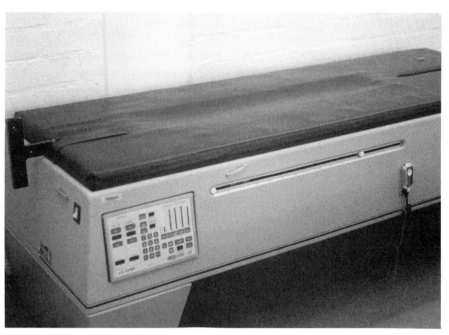

FIGURE 9.7   Intersegmental traction table is used as a form of passive mobility.

men and IVD space. This widening is only temporary and does not permanently alter the dimensions of either structure. The relief gained, however, may be long lasting. The exact mechanism for this relief is not clear but may involve stimulation of mechanoreceptors, improvement of local circulation, and reduction of muscle spasms.

Joint Dysfunction (Hypomobility)

The application of various traction techniques to patients with loss of spinal movement, whether from joint or muscle stiffness, is designed to improve movement, increase circulation to involved areas, and reduce muscle tension.

Certain forms of traction can be regarded as a form of mobilization, because they involve the passive movement of joints by mechanical (*e.g.*, intersegmental traction) or manual (*e.g.*, manual traction) means. Consequently, any condition involving joint hypomobility may respond favorably to traction. One argument against using traction for mobilization is that it is nonspecific and affects many structures simultaneously. With care, however, it may be possible to reduce the effect of such traction forces to a relatively local area of the spine. In addition, manual traction may be useful in the treatment of nonspinal joints. As stated, the use of intersegmental traction provides a very general, but comfortable, mobilization that results in an increase in the movement of spinal structures.

Precautions

Following are some precautions in using spinal traction:

- It should be borne in mind, that traction is usually not the only therapy used. As with other forms of therapy, when it is used the doctor should be alert to changes in the patient's condition that warrant modification in treatment methods. It is particularly important to keep in mind the following rule: *If treatment increases peripheral pain and/or symptoms, it should be discontinued* until both the condition and the therapy have been re-evaluated.

- To minimize any potential injury resulting from inappropriate use of traction (*e.g.,* too much weight or improper patient position), traction should be initiated gently, with progressively increasing force and time as the patient condition warrants.

- Following the application of traction, a patient should be allowed a short rest period before resuming activities. It is not uncommon for patients to feel some pain relief during the application of traction, only to have the relief disappear at the end of the treatment session. It is suggested that the patient should be gradually returned to the upright position to maintain the initial relief.

Contraindications

As with other forms of therapy, spinal traction should be used with care, and the doctor should be aware of conditions or problems that might prevent its use. The following are contraindications to spinal traction:

- structural disease that is secondary to tumor or infection (*e.g.,* osteomyelitis)
- patients with problems that compromise the peripheral vascular system (*e.g.,* diabetes mellitus)
- any condition for which movement is contraindicated (*e.g.,* fractures or dislocations)
- acute stage of joint sprains
- instability
- pregnancy
- osteoporosis and other bone weakening disorders
- patients with a hiatal hernia
- patients with active peptic ulcers
- patients with aortic aneurysms

- patients who are hypertensive
- patients who are claustrophobic
- patients with a recent history of strokes, cerebrovascular accidents, or transient ischemic attacks

Techniques

Lumbar Traction

There is great variation in the methods used to apply traction to the lumbar spine. Traction mode (*e.g.*, sustained or intermittent) depends on both the disorder being treated and on the comfort of the patient. Disc protrusions usually are treated more effectively with sustained traction or with longer hold-rest periods of intermittent traction (60 seconds hold; 20 seconds rest). Joint dysfunction and degenerative disc disease usually respond to shorter hold-rest periods of intermittent traction (30 seconds hold; 10 seconds rest). The following general guidelines are suggested to improve patient acceptance and clinical response:

- The patient must be able to relax. Those patients who are unable to relax may produce enough muscle contraction to actually shorten the spine. It may help to begin a trial treatment with gentle traction forces. These forces may be gradually increased over the course of several treatments as the patient gains confidence in the treatments and in the clinician.
- The harnesses used must be heavy duty and must not slip during treatment. If patients do not feel secure, they almost certainly do not relax. Many of the traction tables use Velcro straps to secure patients to the apparatus. Although these straps are strong enough to hold most forces that may be applied, they often make a noise, as if they are tearing apart. This sound may be discomforting to patients and efforts should be made to reassure them.
- The traction harnesses should be placed next to the skin to reduce slippage.
- All of the slack must be taken up before the traction is initiated. Traction forces should be gradually applied over a period of several minutes. Patients may relax better if they can adapt slowly to the forces.
- Patients should be provided with a hand-held control to stop the traction device if necessary. Although most patients do not use the switch, they usually feel more secure if they have some control.
- I find it helpful to place patients in a lumbar corset following the traction treatment. These devices assist the muscles to support the lower back and provide a measure of security to the patient.

Proper Poundage

To produce a desired effect, the traction force must be great enough to effect a structural change at the spinal segment. Mathews reported separation with 120 pounds of sustained traction for 20 minutes (Mathews, 1968). Others have reported measurable separation in the lumbar spine with forces ranging from 80 to 200 pounds (Cyriax, 1950). A minimal force of one fourth of the patient's body weight is required if a conventional table traction technique is used (Judovich, 1952). A split table will reduce the friction between the patient and the table and should reduce the necessary poundage. It has been shown in cadaver studies that a force of 400 pounds is necessary to produce a rupture of the dorsolumbar spine (DeSeze, Levernieux, 1951).

The following guidelines may be used for the safe and effective application of traction to the lumbar spine:

- begin with approximately 50 pounds
- if the patient improves, continue at the same poundage or increase poundage by 10 pound increments to a maximum of 125 pounds

Patient Position

The patient position, whether prone or supine, and the amount of flexion or extension used depend on the disorder being treated, on the experience of the doctor, on the comfort of the patient, and on the type of equipment being used:

- Saunders suggests treating the patient with disc protrusions in a prone position with a slightly flattened lordosis. He suggests that joint hypomobility and degenerative disc disease are usually more effectively treated with the patient supine and the lumbar spine in a flattened position (Saunders, 1985).

- McElhannon believes the angle of pull of the traction device has a greater impact on the effectiveness of the traction and he places most patients in a supine position (McElhannon, 1984).

- It should be noted that the authors mentioned use different forms of traction tables and their techniques are modified accordingly. It may be that the type of equipment used is the most important aspect in determining the appropriate patient position.

- Patient comfort is important and a trial of manual traction will assist the doctor in determining the most comfortable and the most effective position.

Angle of Pull

The angle of the traction harness pull and the position of the lumbar spine have an impact on the location of the primary traction force. This is most important when using the **Orthion** table (Figure 9.8):

- to treat lumbar conditions the proper angle of pull is between 15 and 50 degrees
- to affect the lower thoracic and upper lumbar segments (L1-L3), the angle of pull must be 15 to 30 degrees
- to affect the lower lumbar segments (L3-L5), the angle of pull must be 30 to 50 degrees
- hypolordosis of the lumbar spine should be treated with an angle of pull from 15 to 30 degrees
- hyperlordosis should be treated with an angle of pull from 30 to 50 degrees

Note: In effect, the lower in the lumbar spine the traction is intended, the greater the angle of pull.

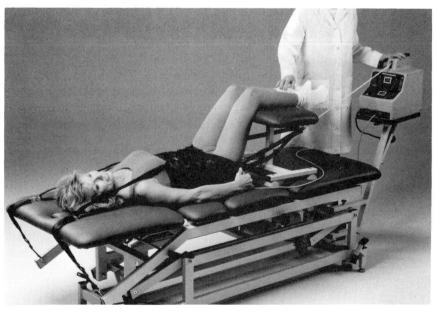

FIGURE 9.8   The angle of pull of the harness is an important factor in localizing the traction effect.

Duration

Traditionally, spinal traction is applied in 20-minute increments. Treatment time may vary depending on the nature of the condition, the type of equipment used, and the response of the patient. The following guidelines are suggested:

- When an intervertebral disc herniation is treated with traction, the treatment time should be short. Of particular importance, the first treatment should only be 3 to 5 minutes in length. This short treatment time allows the clinician to evaluate the patient's response to the traction procedure without undue concern regarding exacerbating the condition. If the patient responds favorably, treatment time may be increased on subsequent visits.
- Although some authors suggest a maximal treatment time of 10 minutes when treating a disc herniation, treatment times may be adjusted to each patient. Treatment times in excess of 20 minutes probably are not wise.
- Joint hypomobility, degenerative disc disease, and joint disease should be treated using a 3 to 1 ratio of hold and rest (30 seconds hold; 10 seconds rest).
- Disc herniations should be treated with a longer hold and rest cycle (60 seconds hold; 20 seconds rest).

Treatment Frequency

As with other forms of therapy, spinal traction has a specific physiologic effect and should be used when that effect is desired. The application of sustained and intermittent traction is usually only warranted for relatively short periods of time:

- daily treatment is suggested for the first 3 days, followed by three times weekly for 2 to 3 weeks
- if traction is to be helpful, some relief should be seen within the first three to five treatments

Unlike other forms of traction, intersegmental traction may be warranted on a continuing basis in some patients. It should not, however, serve as a substitute for stretching and flexibility exercises, nor should it be used as a standard procedure for all patients seen.

Case 1: Lumbar Traction

Joseph R., a 35-year-old executive presents with a history of chronic back pain. The patient states that he injured his back 6 years earlier while snow skiing. Mr. R. relates that after the injury he had a series of unsuccessful treatment by different doctors. He eventually had surgery to remove a herniated lumbar disc. Although the surgery was successful in reducing the extreme back pain, he states that he has had a burning pain in the lower back ever since. Nothing that he has attempted to do has provided any relief for this pain. Recently, the pain has increased and now extends into the right buttock and upper part of the right thigh. Mr. R. does not relate any particular incident or activity with the recent change in his symptoms but does state that he does not wish to have any more surgery.

Evaluation of the patient reveals an apparently healthy, slightly overweight individual who ambulates with some caution. Palpation of the lumbar spine reveals bilateral tenderness in the entire lumbar spine. Tenderness extends to the right gluteal region and along the course of the right sciatic nerve to the posterior aspect of the mid thigh. Orthopedic assessment of the lower back reveals slight stiffness with some loss of flexion and extension. Valsalva maneuver produces an increase in back pain with some radiation into the right thigh. The Achilles tendon reflex is somewhat diminished on the right. All other reflexes and muscle strength are within normal limits. The working diagnosis is chronic lumbar intervertebral disc syndrome with sciatic neuritis.

After discussing treatment options with Mr. R., a trial course of traction is selected in an attempt to reduce the lower back pain. Therapy consists of three treatments per week for 3 weeks. Treatment begins with intermittent traction—using 50 pounds with the patient in a supine position for 8 minutes. If initial traction treatment is tolerated by the patient, 10 pounds will be added with each additional application. Treatment time will be increased by 1 minute every other treatment session. Mr. R. will be provided with a lumbar corset to be worn following the traction treatment. Traction treatment will be accompanied by a stretching program. After the third traction procedure, spinal manipulation will be added to the treatment protocol.

Cervical Traction

Traction to the cervical spine can be applied in the supine position using a traction table. It can also be applied in the seated position, such as with the home (over-door) traction devices. The general guidelines for the safe and effective application of cervical traction are similar to those for traction of the lumbar spine. It is particularly important that patients are able to relax when using cervical traction. In addition, consideration must be given to the effect of the traction device on the temporomandibular (TM) joint. Because most cervical traction devices place some pressure on the TM apparatus, patients with problems in this joint may be adversely affected by the application of cervical traction.

Proper Poundage

As with lumbar traction, in order to produce a desired effect the traction force must be great enough to effect a structural change at the spinal segment. For obvious reasons, much less force is required in the cervical region:

- forces of 25 to 45 pounds are necessary to produce measurable changes in the posterior structures (Judovich, 1952).
- the maximal force should not exceed 45 pounds.
- forces of 120 pounds have been shown to be necessary to cause a disc rupture at the C5-C6 level (DeSeze and Lervernieux, 1951).
- it has been shown that a traction force of only 10 pounds will pro-duce separation of the atlanto-axial joints; consequently, less force is necessary when the upper cervical spine is the target area (Daugh-erty and Erhard, 1977).
- some studies have shown a compression or narrowing of the cervical joint space with cervical traction; this has been attributed to muscle tension and guarding and it is imperative that the patient relax for traction to be effective.

For the safe and effective application of traction to the cervical spine:

- it is suggested that the doctor begin with a traction force of between 10 and 15 pounds
- if the patient improves, continue at the same poundage or increase poundage by 5-pound increments to a maximum of 45 pounds.

Patient Position

When cervical traction is applied using a table type of apparatus, the patient is usually in a supine position (Figure 9.9). The position of the cervical spine will have a direct effect on the location of the traction effect:

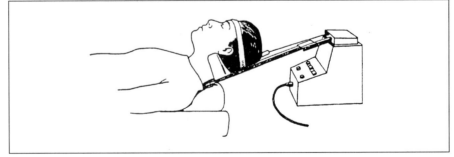

FIGURE 9.9   As with other forms of traction, the position of the cervical spine has a direct effect on the location of the traction effect.

- If the head is allowed to lay on the table with the cervical spine in a neutral or extended position, the traction will exert its maximal effect on the anterior intervertebral structures such as the intervertebral disc. When the objective is separation of the interbody joints, the patient should be positioned in such a neutral or extended position.

- If the head is maintained in a flexed, forward-bent position, the traction will exert its maximal effect on the posterior structures, such as the facet articulations and the intervertebral foramen. When the objective is separation of the posterior articulations, the patient should be positioned with the neck in a flexed position.

- The greater the angle of flexion, the lower in the cervical spine is the area affected by the traction force. The position of the head and neck can be adjusted to ensure that separation occurs at the desired location. This is most easily accomplished by communicating with the patient during the initial application. The best position is the one that localizes the traction force in the area of pain.

When the over-door apparatus is used, the patient is typically seated. The position of the cervical spine can be modified by altering the position of the chair and by turning the patient either to face toward or away from the apparatus (Figure 9.10). The patient should be moved until the traction exerts an effect wherein it creates the most relief. There is no substitute for trial and error in establishing the most appropriate position for the patient and the traction device.

Angle of Pull

The angle of pull of the traction harness will influence the area affected by the traction device:

- it is suggested that an angle of 0 to 15 degrees be used for the upper cervical spine.

- the angle should be increased by 5-degree increments for each progressively lower cervical segment.

- both the angle of pull and the position of the head have a similar effect in changing the location of the traction forces.

Duration

The duration for cervical traction should follow the same guidelines as those listed for lumbar traction. Patients who use the cervical over-the-door devices at home should be instructed to limit each treatment time to no more than 15 minutes.

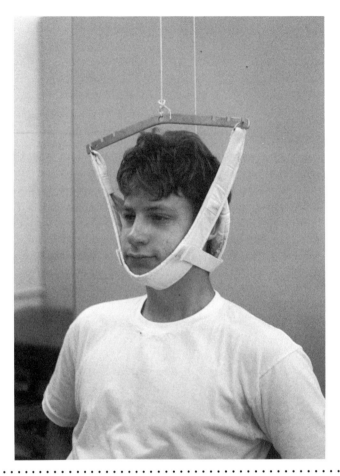

FIGURE 9.10   When an over-the-door apparatus is used, the patient typically is seated.

Frequency

The frequency of cervical traction that is performed in a clinical setting should follow the same guidelines as those listed for lumbar traction. The application of cervical traction with a home over-the-door device can be more frequent and can be a helpful and cost-effective form of therapy for patients with stressful lives and chronic conditions. Treatment frequency may be adjusted on an as needed basis.

Case 2: Cervical Traction

John T., a 55-year-old high school principal, presents with a history of chronic neck pain and muscle tension headaches. The patient states that he has had problems for many years and has basically learned to live with them. He relates using medication to control his pain. He expresses concern that he must continually increase the amount of medication needed to control the pain. His job is particularly stressful and he sometimes feels that he may have to take an early retirement because of his condition. He has had a variety of treatments over the years, including different forms of physical therapy. Although the treatments have provided some temporary relief, nothing has been successful at controlling the pain over the long term.

Evaluation reveals marked tenderness to palpation in the cervical spine accompanied by muscle tension bilaterally throughout the neck and upper back. Range of motion of the cervical spine is limited and accompanied by pain in all directions. Compression increases the cervical discomfort, whereas manual distraction of the head yields a slight reduction in pain. Reflexes and muscle strength are essentially normal. Radiographs of the cervical spine reveal moderate degenerative changes in the cervical spine with some evidence of disc thinning at the C5-6 and C6-7 levels. Osteophyte formation, which is present in the lower cervical spine, is most marked at the C5-6 level. Diagnosis is (1) chronic cervicalgia with degenerative joint disease of the cervical spine and (2) cervicogenic headaches.

The treatment regimen suggested consists of:

- visits 1 through 3: electrical stimulation to relieve spasm of the cervical muscles, gentle grade II mobilization of the cervical spine, manual traction of the neck using a towel, and relaxation exercises
- visit 4: continue with electrical stimulation, increase from grade II mobilization procedure to spinal manipulation (grade V), continue with manual traction, fit patient with home cervical traction device, and instruct on home treatment technique
- visits 5 through 10: electrical stimulation, spinal manipulation, manual traction, range of motion exercises for the cervical spine
- additional visits: discontinue electrical stimulation, continue with spinal manipulation, manual traction, and exercises

References and Suggested Reading

Cox J. Low back pain. Baltimore: Williams and Wilkins, 1992.

Cyriax J. Treatment of lumbar disc lesions. Br Med J 1950;2:1434-1438.

Daugherty R, Erhard R. Segmentalized cervical traction. Proceedings, International Federation of Orthopedic Manipualtive Therapists, Kent B (ed). Vail, Colorado, 1977 pp 189-195.

DeSeze S, Levernieux J. Les tractions vertebrales. Semaine des Hopitaux (Paris) 1951;27:2075.

Gupta R, Ramarao S. Epidurography in reduction of lumbar disc prolapse by traction. Arch Phys Med Rehabil 1978;59:322-327.

Judovich B. Herniated cervical disc. Am J Surg 1952;84:649.

Judovich B. Lumbar traction therapy. JAMA 1955;159:549.

Mathews J. Dynamic discography: a study of lumbar traction. Arch Phys Med Rehabil 1968;9:275-279.

McKenzie RA. The lumbar spine: mechanical diagnosis and therapy. Waikane, New Zealand: Spinal Publications, 1981.

McElhannon JE, A guide to physio-therapeutics. Anaheim Hills, CA: McElhannon, 1984, pp 11-17.

Natchev E. A manual on auto-traction treatment for low back pain. E. Natcher, Sweden, 1984.

Saunders HD. Evaluation, treatment and prevention of musculoskeletal disorders. H Duane Saunders, 1985.

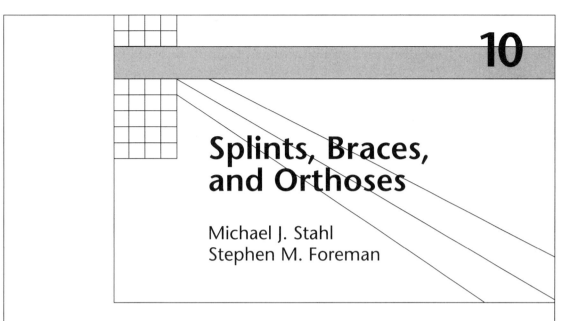

10

Splints, Braces, and Orthoses

Michael J. Stahl
Stephen M. Foreman

Learning Objectives

At the completion of this chapter, you should be able to:

1. Understand the general purposes of supports and devices.
2. Determine when the use of orthopedic supports or braces is appropriate.
3. Select the most suitable splints, braces, and orthoses for conditions commonly encountered in the chiropractic office.

*Private practice, Woodland Hills, California

As the chiropractic profession enters its second century, Doctors of Chiropractic in today's clinical environment have available an expanded range of treatment methods that were not available to our predecessors. Not only have we as professionals established that we can help patients by detecting and treating subluxations, we also have provided great relief in our diagnosis and treatment of industrial injuries, personal injuries, and many sports injuries. Along with the growth of our patient base, there has developed a need for adjuncts, such as therapy and braces, to chiropractic manipulative therapy (CMT).

The correct application or use of orthopedic supports, braces, and orthoses lends itself to our patient base quite well. Not all braces available in the general marketplace are used by chiropractors. As a general rule we do not treat fractures, dislocations, and frank neurologic deficits; therefore, topics such as casts, halo braces, Denis Browne splints, and so forth, will not be discussed in this chapter. However, soft tissue injuries, such as lumbar strains, tennis elbow complaints, shoulder injuries, and heel spurs, have very little potential morbidity, and thus they are well suited to effective treatment in today's chiropractic office.

Most of the supports and devices used in the chiropractic office can serve one or more of the four general purposes listed below.

General Purposes

Anatomic Support (ex, soft cervical collar, w/t acute conditions for support)

In acute stage usually

Support of injured anatomic structures can be valuable in speeding healing and in reducing inflammation that arises from excessive motion. A common example of this type of anatomic support is the soft cervical collar used following an auto accident. Although such devices are not mandatory in every such injury, in those that are moderate to severe in nature, they can produce great relief for the injured patient.

Injury Prevention (knee supports w/ stays, rib pads)

After the injuries have reached their maximal point of physiologic healing, supports, splints, or braces can be used to prevent undesirable or excessive motions (*e.g.*, knee supports with metal stays prevent lateral deviation and potential injury to the medial collateral ligaments).

Other specialized devices have been developed to prevent injury in delicate anatomic areas which may be exposed to higher than normal forces due to occupational or recreational endeavors. Two examples of this type of device are the protective rib pads used by the quarterback in football games and the throat protector that hangs from the bottom of the catcher's mask in baseball.

³ *Therapeutic or Anatomic Correction* (*patellar brace*)

Some braces or supports can provide anatomic correction by preventing aberrant anatomic motion in certain areas. A good example of this is the patellar brace used in patients with patellar tracking conditions. This type of brace holds the patella in proper alignment and allows it to track without the potential for dislocation.

⁴ *Anatomic Stabilization* (*rigid/semi-rigid orthotics*)

Some orthopedic supports or braces are used for anatomic foundational support. One prime example is rigid or semi-rigid shoe orthotics. These hold the arch of the foot in proper alignment despite the effects of weight and gravity on the arch of the foot.

It is important for the clinician to be cognizant of the potential uses of various braces and supports to achieve the desired clinical effect. The use of orthopedic supports and braces will have to be planned with some thought as to the timing of the proper use. Just as the application of a plaster cast over a fracture 4 months postinjury would have little clinical benefit, braces and supports must also be used at the proper time.

Acute Phase

The most commonly encountered need for supports in the chiropractic office arises when a patient presents in the acute phase of injury. Normally, a traumatic event causes inflammation in the affected tissues. This is usually a byproduct of the traumatized tissues and the cellular response to repair in the injured tissues. During the acute phase, an injured muscle will respond with a protective reflex known as "muscle splinting," or "muscle guarding." With this comes the inability of the muscles to perform their normal physiologic functions and the application of a support helps break this reflex cycle. As seen in the cervical spine example, paraspinal muscles primarily support the head and control motion of the spine. When these supporting muscles are injured and fail to support the head and spine, the need for a cervical collar becomes quite obvious.

Clinical assessment after the traumatic event allows the doctor to determine the severity of injuries and, therefore, the clinical need for such a support. Mild injuries usually have minimal need for such a device. If support is indicated, the general goal is to allow the maximal amount of prudent motion and the least amount of immobilization possible (*e.g.*, a plaster cast is not necessary for a mild lumbar strain, as this is immobilization overkill for such a benign condition).

The degree of immobilization and support, therefore, is dictated by the degree of injury. Another example, a non-displaced cervical compression fracture would be best served by a Philadelphia collar, whereas a cervical strain injury, which would not necessitate such a rigid support, would be more properly treated with a soft collar.

The other primary function of the correctly used orthopedic support is timing. As soon as tissues have been traumatized, healing begins at the cellular level. The cellular response and healing activity is greatest during the acute stages of the injury. It is the cellular response that produces the cardinal signs of swelling, reddening of the area, and increased warmth. During this initial physiologic response, the healing process can be compromised with excessive motion, thus, the need for a brace or support. In a grade I collateral knee sprain, the ligaments have not been compromised to a degree that affects the integrity of the joint. However, in such an injury, excessive motions can undermine the healing of the ligaments and their attempt to return to normal.

In the following pages various supports, orthoses, and braces are discussed in regard to anatomic areas, and issues surrounding their proper use. These represent some of the more commonly encountered conditions and braces seen in the chiropractic office.

Anatomic Applications

Foot

Heel Cups (heel spurs or plantar fasciitis)

caused by abnormal tractioning

- Commonly used for: heel spurs or plantar fascitis
- Diagnostic testing findings: x-ray, heel spurs
- Examination indications: pain on palpating heel
- History indications: pain during running, aerobics, prolonged walking
- Contraindications: none
- Student notes:

Heel Lifts (structural or functional short legs)

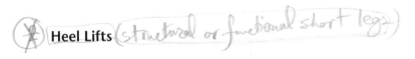

- Commonly used with: structural or functional short legs
- Diagnostic testing indication: x-ray, leg length discrepancy
- Examination indications: short leg, functional or structural

- History indications: scoliosis
- Contraindications: hip and knee degeneration, moderate to severe; genu varus or valgus deformities
- Student notes:

✕ Soft Orthotics (foot pronation)

- Commonly used with: foot pronation
- Diagnostic testing indications: none
- Examination indications: various
- History indications: foot pain; chronic low back pain
- Contraindications: none
- Student notes:

Ankle

Ⓧ Soft Compressive (Elastic) Braces (Grade I ankle sprains)

- Commonly used with: grade I ankle sprains (Figure 10.1)
- Diagnostic testing indications: x-ray
- Examination indications: decreased range of motion, swelling, negative drawer signs
- History indications: pain after traumatic inversion or eversion
- Contraindications: brace placed too tight, prevents circulation
- Student notes:

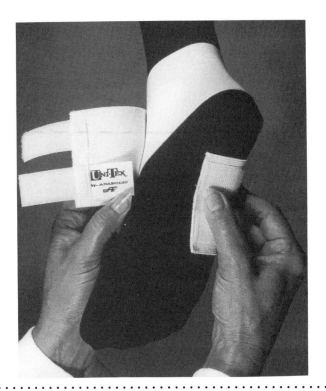

FIGURE 10.1   An elastic or compression ankle support being applied.

⊗ Hard Brace—Prevents Excessive Inversion or Eversion

(grade II ankles sprains awaiting for surgical opinion)

- Commonly used with: grade II ankle sprains, waiting for surgical opinion
- Diagnostic testing indications: x-ray, possible computerized tomography (CT) or magnetic resonance imaging (MRI) evaluations
- Examination indications: swelling, eccymosis, positive drawer's sign, decreased range of motion
- History indications: possible long history of prior inversion or eversion ankle sprains
- Contraindications: fractures of ankle mortise, compromised vascular status secondary to excessive compression
- Student notes:

Knee

✳ Soft Brace (General Support) *(Grade I MCL/LCL, sprain)*

- Commonly used with: grade I medial or lateral collateral ligament sprain; muscular strains (Figures 10.2—10.4)
- Diagnostic testing indications: x-ray, MRI

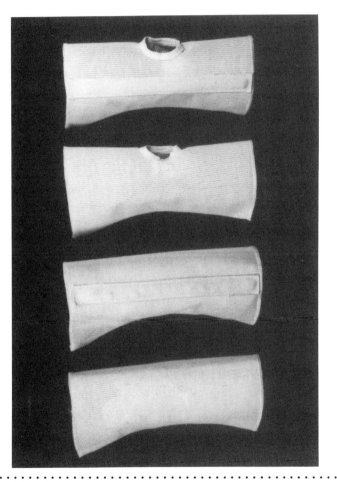

FIGURE 10.2 Side views of four different knee supports. The bottom support is soft and compressive without an access panel for the patella. The second support from the bottom is the same elastic support with a semirigid rod support on the medial and lateral side for support in those directions. The third support from the bottom is an elastic support with an opening for the patella. This provides some additional support in this area. The final support or brace is the compression brace with semirigid supports on the medial and lateral side.

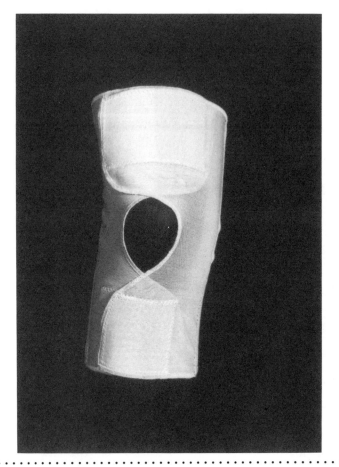

FIGURE 10.3   Front view of a soft support with Velcro closures. This allows the patient to vary the amount of compression to the joint.

- Examination indications: negative stability tests, negative drawer's sign, decreased range of motion, swelling
- History indications: traumatically induced valgus or varus motions
- Contraindications: grade II or III sprains, fractures, anterior cruciate ligament (ACL) sprains
- Student notes:

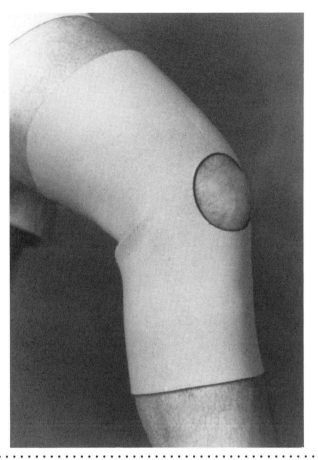

FIGURE 10.4   Neoprene open patellar knee sleeve. Designed to give gentle support to the knee with greater mobility to the patella.

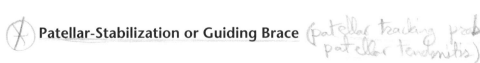

Patellar-Stabilization or Guiding Brace (patellar tracking probs, patellar tendonitis)

- Commonly used with: patellar tracking disorders, jumper's knee, patellar tendonitis (Figure 10.5)
- Diagnostic testing indications: MRI, CT, x-ray (sunrise view)
- Examination indications: crepitus, swelling
- History indications: pain when climbing stairs; pain after strenuous athletic activities
- Contraindications: none

• Student notes:

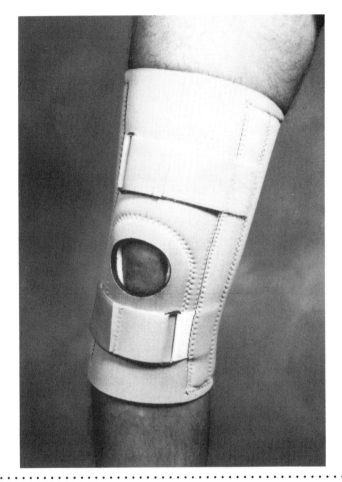

FIGURE 10.5   Neoprene patellar knee support. The Velcro closures, medial and lateral stays, and patella support allows maximal immobilization to the patella.

⊕ Prevention of Excessive Lateral Flexion (Grade I/II, MCL/LCL sprains)

- Commonly used with: grade I (possibly II) medial and lateral collateral ligament sprain; placement awaiting surgical opinion
- Diagnostic testing indications: x-ray, CT, MRI
- Examination indications: positive stability testing
- History indications: traumatically induced varus or valgus stresses
- Contraindications: fractures
- Student notes:

⊕ Prevention of Excessive Rotation Braces (post ACL repair)

- Commonly used: after ACL surgical repair
- Diagnostic testing indications: MRI
- Examination indications: surgical repair of ACL
- History indications: past history of ACL injury, surgical intervention
- Contraindications: incorrect diagnosis
- Student notes:

Coccyx

Doughnut

- Commonly used with: coccyxdynia
- Diagnostic testing indications: x-ray
- Examination indications: pain on palpation
- History indications: possible pain on defecation; history of trauma (*e.g.,* falling on ice)

- Contraindications: avascular necrosis of distal segment of coccyx
- Student notes:

Lumbar Spine

Soft Brace (S/S injuries)

- Commonly used with: sprain or strain injuries (Figure 10.6)
- Diagnostic testing indications: negative x-rays
- Examination indications: decreased range of motion, muscle spasms
- History indications: various
- Contraindications: fractures
- Student notes:

Soft Brace with Rigid Stays (IVDS, noncompromising compression fx's)

- Commonly used with: intervertebral disc syndrome (IVDS), noncompromising compression fractures, severe sprain injuries (Figure 10.7)
- Diagnostic testing indications: x-ray, CT, MRI
- Examination indications: relief with traction, IVF compression signs, nerve root tension signs (straight leg raising [SLR], Braggard's sign)
- History indications: various
- Contraindications: cauda equina syndrome
- Student notes:

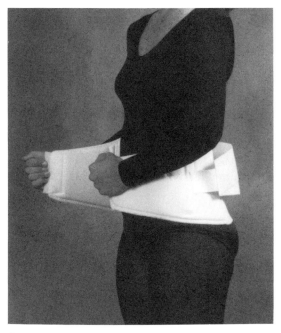

A

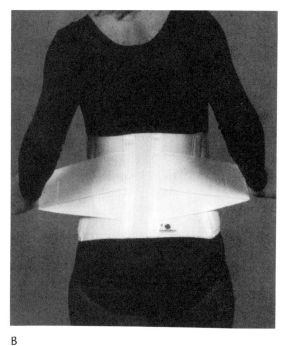

B

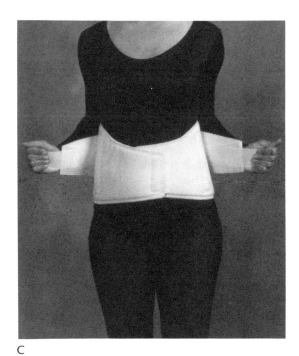

C

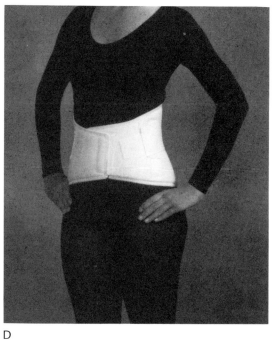

D

· ·

FIGURE 10.6   Application of the soft lumbar support. **A.** The initial overlapping of the front section with a Velcro closure. **B, C.** The side panels being pulled tightly after which they fasten to the front of the belt. **D.** The soft lumbar support once it has been properly applied.

⚹ **Rigid or Hard Brace** (IVDS)

- Commonly used with: IVDS
- Diagnostic testing indications: x-ray
- Examination indications: mild sensory loss, mild motor loss, relief with traction, IVF signs, nerve root tension signs (SLR, Braggards), intrathecal signs (Valsava's maneuver, Naffiziger's syndrome)
- History indications: radiating pain into lower extremity possible; traumatic event
- Contraindications: various
- Student notes:

⚹ **Body Cast** (Compression fx's moderate/severe lumbar discopathy)

- Commonly used with: compression fractures, moderate or severe lumbar discopathy
- Diagnostic testing indications: MRI, CT, electromyograph (EMG), nerve conduction velocity (NCV)
- Examination indications: possible (mild) motor, sensory or reflex deficits; positive nerve root tension testing; positive intrathecal signs
- History indications: lower back pain with a dermatomal distribution of pain or numbness (usually past the knee) intensified by coughing, sneezing, straining on defecation
- Contraindications: cauda equina syndrome; motor, sensory, reflex deficits that are not mild
- Student notes:

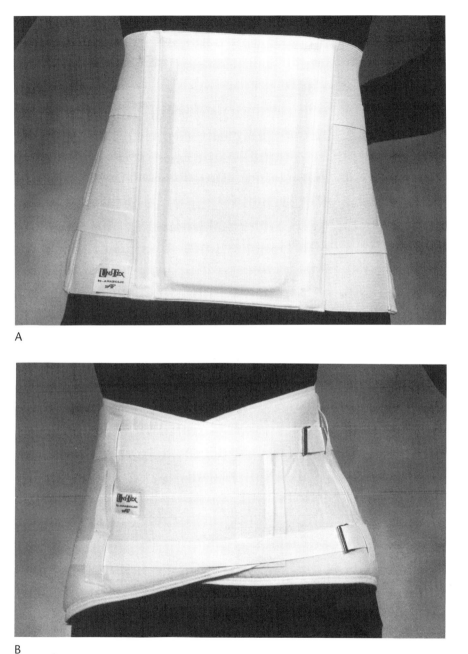

A

B

FIGURE 10.7 **A.** Back view of a lumbar/sacroiliac support with a rigid stay. These are quite similiar to the soft lumbar support, but the rigid plastic stay insert can be softened by heat and molded to the patient's low back. Once inserted into the support it provides additional immobilization. **B.** Front view of same support. Note the lower position which allows support of the sacroiliac joints.

Thoracic Spine and Ribs

Figure 8 Brace *(clavicular fx's, mild AC seperations)*

- Commonly used with: clavicular fractures, acromioclavicular (AC) separations (mild)
- Diagnostic testing indications: x-ray
- Examination indications: see x-ray
- History indications: usually a history of some type of trauma
- Contraindications: incorrect diagnosis
- Student notes:

Rib Belt *(non-displaced rib fx's)*

- Commonly used with: nondisplaced rib fractures, pleurisy, or intercostal neuralgia (Figure 10.8)
- Diagnostic testing indications: x-ray
- Examination indications: pain on inspiration, sneezing, coughing
- History indications: acute onset following blunt trauma; painful coughing, sneezing
- Contraindications: pneumothorax
- Student notes:

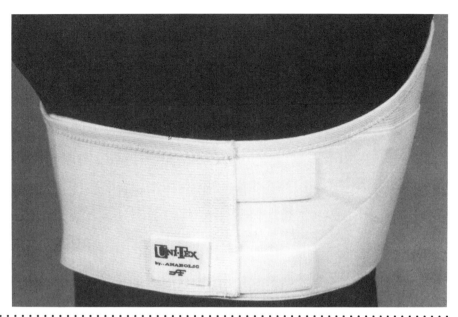

FIGURE 10.8   Front view of a rib belt for female patients.

Cervical Spine

Soft Collar (S/s, tortocollis, whiplash)

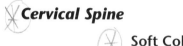

- Commonly used with: muscle strains, torticollis, cervical acceleration/deceleration (CAD) injuries (Figure 10.9)

- Diagnostic testing indications: x-ray, rule out fractures, ligamentous injuries

- Examination indications: foraminal compression signs, relief of pain on cervical distraction

- History indications: various

- Contraindications: incorrect diagnosis; prolonged use can lead to dependency and atrophy

- Student notes:

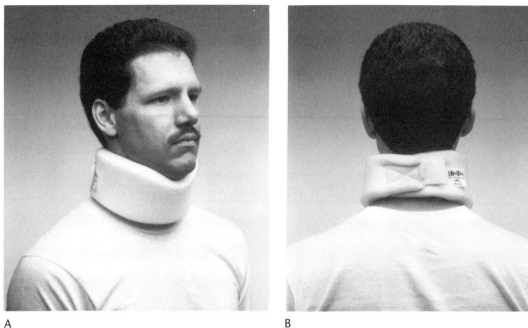

A   B

FIGURE 10.9   **A.** Front view of a cervical collar. The notch in the collar allows space for the chin. **B.** Back view of the soft cervical collar.

 Philadelphia Brace *(mild compression fx's, avulsion fx's, clay-shoveler's fx)*

- Commonly used with: mild compression fractures, avulsion fractures or ligamentous tearing, clay-shoveler's fracture (possible)(Figure 10.10)
- Diagnostic testing indications: x-ray, CT, MRI
- Examination indications: defer to diagnostic test results
- History indications: history of trauma; in spontaneous injuries of this nature, suspect pathologic fractures
- Contraindications: incorrect diagnosis
- Student notes:

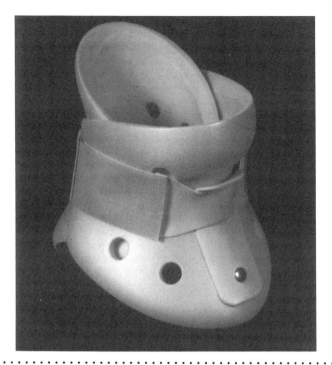

FIGURE 10.10   Philadephia rigid cervical collar. These lightweight collars are made from foam and plastic and can be shaped to conform to the patient. Closure is maintained by a Velcro strap.

Shoulders

 Sling

- Commonly used with: bursitis, tendonitis, strains, AC separations (mild), rotator cuff injuries (mild) (Figure 10.11)
- Diagnostic testing indications: x-ray, MRI
- Examination indications: Codman's sign, defer to history and diagnostic testing
- History indications: various
- Contraindications: prolonged use can lead to adhesive capsulitis, which can lead to a more ominous clinical future than the original presenting injuries
- Student notes:

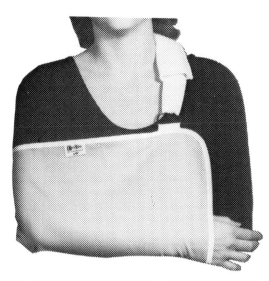

FIGURE 10.11   Soft cloth arm sling is used to support the arm and take pressure off of the shoulder.

Sling with Anti-abduction

- Commonly used with: anterior dislocation
- Diagnostic testing indications: x-ray, MRI
- Examination indications: defer to diagnostic testing; history; possible positive apprehension test
- History indications: either single traumatic event or recurrent history of dislocations; in such conditions look for "hatchet" and Hill-Sachs defect, Bankart lesions, or fractures on x-rays, which can be signs of long-term instability of the joint
- Contraindications: chronic dislocations; adhesive capsulitis
- Student notes:

Elbow

Soft Compressive Supports

- Commonly used with: mild bursitis; strain injuries (Figure 10.12)
- Diagnostic testing indications: none

- Examination indications: tenderness on palpation; inflammation of bursa
- History indications: history of overuse; repetitive trauma
- Contraindications: none
- Student notes:

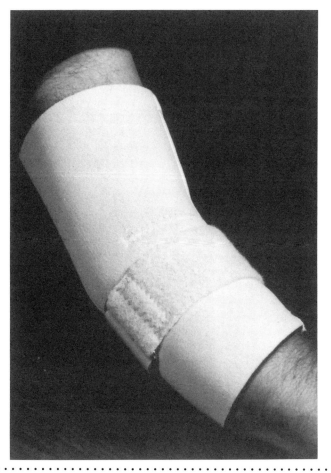

FIGURE 10.12   This elbow support model is desgned as a soft compression sleeve; it is made of neoprene and features a Velcro compression band.

Tennis Elbow and Forearm Compressive Bands

- Commonly used with: tennis elbow, golfer's elbow (Figure 10.13)
- Diagnostic testing indications: none
- Examination indications: tenderness at insertion of wrist extensors; positive Mill's test
- History indications: avid tennis player or golfer
- Contraindications: none
- Student notes:

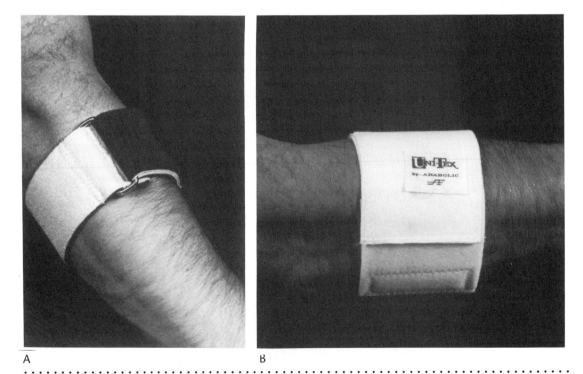

A   B

FIGURE 10.13   **A.** Neoprene tennis elbow strap. Provides support and compression to the local area. **B.** Elastic version of tennis elbow wrap.

Wrist

Soft Compressive

- Commonly used with: strain injuries (Figure 10.14)
- Diagnostic testing indications: none
- Examination indications: various
- History indications: relief when doing repetitive tasks
- Contraindications: none
- Student notes:

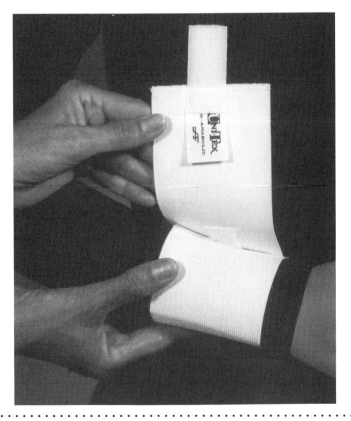

FIGURE 10.14 Elastic wrist compression band.

Cock-up Splint (carpal tunnel)

- Commonly used with: carpal tunnel syndrome (Figure 10.15)
- Diagnostic testing indications: EMG (possible)
- Examination indications: possible positive Tinel's and Phalen's signs
- History indications: repetitive recreational or occupational endeavors using the hand
- Contraindications: incorrect diagnosis; progressive neurologic deficits
- Student notes:

Finger

Sugar Tongue Splints (sprains)

- Commonly used with: mild sprains
- Diagnostic testing indications: x-ray
- Examination indications: decreased range of motion, swelling
- History indications: recent single trauma
- Contraindications: incorrect diagnosis
- Student notes:

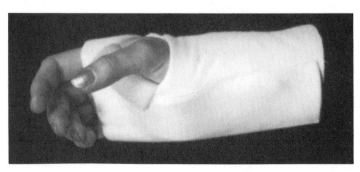

FIGURE 10.15   Cock-up splint with rigid stay. The Velcro closer allows variable compression to the wrist.

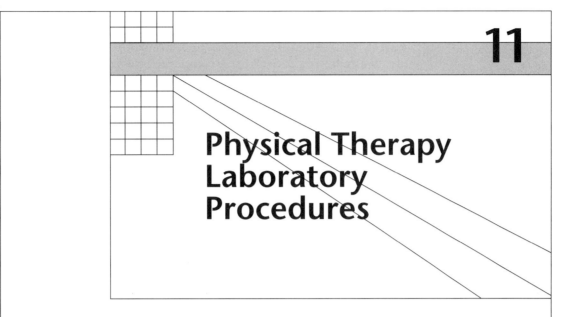

Physical Therapy Laboratory Procedures

Learning Objectives

At the completion of this chapter, you should be able to:

1. Use the techniques involved in the clinical application of the procedures.
2. Determine when the modalities are properly or improperly applied.
3. Understand the procedures from both the doctor's and the patient's perspective.

This section of the text is designed as a guide to assist the student gain experience with the use of the various physical modalities that have been presented. It is suggested that each of the lessons provided be completed by students attempting to learn the techniques involved in the clinical application of the procedures. One of the most important aspects of these exercises is to provide first-hand knowledge of what the patient will experience when the modalities are properly, or improperly applied. Consequently, it is suggested that students go through each of the procedures in pairs. Each person should alternate between doctor and patient. Students should perform the procedure on their laboratory partner and should have the procedure performed on themselves. There is no substitute for first-hand experience.

The purpose of this laboratory section is to familiarize the student with each of the methods and materials used to increase or decrease the temperature of the various tissues.

Thermal Modalities

Cryotherapy

Ice Packs

Take an ice pack from the freezer and wrap it in a clean, dry towel. Place the ice pack on the lower back or the ankle and leave it in contact for 15 minutes. Describe the sensation(s) experienced in order of occurrence and record the time at which the feeling changes from one sensation to the next:

Sensation/time: _____

Sensation/time: _____

Sensation/time: _____

Sensation/time: _____

It is helpful to experiment with all of the various application techniques to appreciate the differences between them. The various applications of cryotherapy include commercial ice packs, ice cubes in a plastic bag, and ice applied directly to the skin. Each has a slightly different intensity and, consequently, a different patient response.

Ice Massage

Fill several styrofoam cups approximately one half full of water and place each of the cups in the freezer. After allowing the water to freeze completely, take one of the styrofoam cups from the freezer and remove the bottom 1 inch of the cup. Invert the cup and use the remaining styrofoam as an insulated handle. Apply the ice directly to the skin over the knee joint of a lab partner. Move the ice cup in a slow, circular motion over the knee. Describe the sensation(s) that are experienced and record the time at which the feeling changes. Repeat the same procedure in a different location such as the lower back, neck, and upper back:

Sensation/time: _____

Sensation/time: _____

Sensation/time: _____

Sensation/time: _____

Ice Massage/Stretch
Use the ice cup to reduce the pain and dysfunction resulting from a myofascial trigger point (TP). Identify a myofascial trigger point (upper trapezius or levator scapulae). Evaluate the length of the muscle containing the trigger point. Place the ice cup over the TP and rotate the cup slowly over the skin for a short period of time, approximately 20 seconds. Remove the cup and set it aside. Stretch the muscle using a postisometric or postcontraction stretch procedure. Repeat the procedure several times. Re-evaluate the muscle length and note any difference that has occurred.

Superficial Heat

Paraffin Bath
Place your hand, up to the wrist, in a paraffin bath and remove it immediately. The paraffin should coat your entire hand and wrist. As soon as the paraffin has cooled sufficiently to allow it to harden (just a few seconds), dip your hand in the bath again and remove. Repeat this process 8 to 10 times allowing a thick layer of paraffin to coat your hand and wrist. Wrap the hand in plastic wrap and then in a clean, dry towel. Keep the hand wrapped for 20 minutes and describe the sensation(s) that you experience:

Sensation/time: _____

Sensation/time: _____

Sensation/time: _____

Note: Be sure to remove any jewelry (*i.e.*, rings and watches) before using the paraffin bath.

Moist Heat (Hydrocollator)
Place your lab partner in a prone position on a therapy table and lay several layers of clean, dry toweling on the lower back. Take a moist heat pack from the hydrocollator unit and wrap it in a terry cloth cover. Place the cover on

the towels and leave it in position for 20 minutes. Periodically, lift the hydrocollator pack and observe the changes that take place on the patient's skin. Record your observations. Ask the patient to record the sensation(s) experienced and record these observations:

Sensation/time: _____

Sensation/time: _____

Sensation/time: _____

Infrared Lamps

Place your lab partner in a prone position on the therapy table and expose the skin of the lower back. Place the infrared lamp approximately 18 inches from the skin and leave in place for 20 minutes. Observe and record the changes that take place:

Sensation/time: _____

Sensation/time: _____

Sensation/time: _____

Note: Be sure to remove any metal such as belts and bra straps before using the infrared lamp.

Deep Heat

Shortwave Diathermy

Place your lab partner in a prone position on the therapy table and expose the skin of the lower back. Place a clean, dry towel on the skin. Place the **autotherm** drum next to the skin and turn on the timer to 15 minutes. Raise the intensity until the patient feels a gentle warming sensation and adjust the tuner to the patient's resonance.

Repeat the above procedure using the **pulsatherm** by placing the pad electrodes on either side of the lumbar spine. Set the timer at 15 minutes and raise the intensity until the patient feels a gentle warming. Observe and record the feelings experienced during the treatment:

Sensation/time: _____

Sensation/time: _____

Sensation/time: _____

Note: Be sure to remove any metal such as belts and bra straps before using the diathermy. It is also helpful to remove contact lenses when using shortwave diathermy.

Evaluate the length of the hamstring muscles bilaterally. Place your lab partner in a prone position on the therapy table. Expose the skin over the hamstrings and place a clean, dry towel on the skin. Locate the **autotherm** drum next to the skin over one of the muscles and turn on the timer to 15 minutes. Raise the intensity until the patient feels a gentle warming sensation and adjust the tuner to the patient's resonance. After the application, re-evaluate the hamstring length and compare to that noted prior to heating.

Note: The application of deep heat prior to stretching may be one of the best uses of this form of passive modality.

Therapeutic Ultrasound

Although the application of therapeutic ultrasound has many effects, it is typically used to increase the temperature of the deeper tissues, particularly the ligaments and tendons near the bone.

The following parameters are suggested for ultrasound:

Condition	Thin Tissue	Thick Tissue
Acute condition		
duty cycle	pulsed	pulsed
intensity	0.5-1.0 w/cm^2	1.0-1.5 w/cm^2
time	4-6 minutes	4-6 minutes
Chronic condition		
duty cycle	continuous	continuous
intensity	1.0-1.5 w/cm^2	1.5-2.0 w/cm^2
time	6-8 minutes	6-8 minutes

Note: If ultrasound is used underwater, add 0.5 w/cm^2 to the intensity setting.

Place your lab partner in a seated position on the therapy table and expose the shoulder. Apply some coupling agent to the skin over the shoulder and to the surface of the ultrasound transducer head (be careful not to get any gel on the patient's clothing or in his or her hair). Before you turn on the power to the ultrasound, practice the movement of the sound head. You can either rotate the sound head slowly in concentric overlapping circles or in longitudinal overlapping strokes. Be sure to keep the sound head in contact with the patient's skin and in continual motion during the course of the treatment. It is not necessary to move the sound head rapidly, simply continually.

Chronic Shoulder Pain (Supraspinatus Tendinitis). Determine the clinical problems you might encounter, the therapeutic objectives you would have, and what parameters you would use for a patient with chronic shoulder pain:

Clinical problems: _____

_____

_____

Therapeutic objectives: _____   _____

_____

_____

Parameters:

duty cycle _____ intensity _____

time _____

Describe the sensation(s) that you experience:

Sensation/time: _____

Sensation/time: _____

Acute Lower Back Sprain. Determine the clinical problems you might encounter, the therapeutic objectives you would have, and what parameters you would use for a patient with a recent lower back sprain:

Clinical problems: _____

_____

_____

Therapeutic objectives: _____

_____

_____

Parameters:

duty cycle _____ intensity _____

time _____

Note: When you are done with the treatment, take time to clean the patient with a towel and wipe the coupling gel from the head of the ultrasound unit.

Chronic Wrist Pain (Healed Fracture)—Underwater Application. Determine what clinical problems you might encounter, the therapeutic objectives you would have, and what parameters you would select for a patient with a chronic wrist problem:

Clinical problems: _____

_____

_____

Therapeutic objectives: _____

_____

_____

Parameters:

duty cycle _____ intensity _____

time _____

Myofascial Trigger Points. Determine what clinical problems you might encounter, the therapeutic objectives you would have, and what parameters you would select for a patient with myofascial trigger points in the upper trapezius muscle:

Clinical problems: _____

_____

_____

Therapeutic objectives: _____

_____

_____

Parameters:

duty cycle _____ intensity _____

time _____

Note: As with other treatments that are directed at myofascial trigger points, it is important to follow the application of ultrasound with a stretching procedure.

Electrical Stimulation

To learn to use electrical stimulation in a clinical setting, it is first necessary to become familiar with the equipment that is used and with the physiologic responses to changes in parameters. The following laboratory exercises are designed to begin the task of familiarizing the student with the various types of electrical stimulation devices. At first glance, each of the stimulation devices may look significantly different and the task of identifying and using each of them may appear intimidating. If we initially focus on the differences between the devices, they may indeed be confusing. If, instead, we focus on the similarities between them, the task is relatively straight forward.

To simplify, we will divide the task of learning to use the electrical stimulation devices into three separate sections: (1) becoming familiar with the equipment, (2) experimenting with the various controls, and (3) practice setting up treatment protocols. The first exercise is designed to familiarize students with all of the various electrical stimulation devices that are available. It is helpful to have several different stimulation devices available to note some of the similarities and differences.

Electrical Stimulation Laboratory Exercise #1: Familiarizing Yourself with Electrical Stimulation Devices

Position yourself at any of the electrical stimulators and identify the type of electrical stimulation device that you will be using. Hint: if you see a polarity switch, a dispersive pad, or a volt meter, the machine is a high-voltage generator (HVG). If you see a frequency control that uses the term "beat frequency" and a mode switch that uses the terms "quadpolar or premodulated," you have an interferential unit. If none of these features are present, you probably are using a low-voltage, alternating current, sine wave stimulator.

Next, identify the following controls: (1) the power switch, (2) the starter button or control, (3) the timer, (4) the frequency control, (5) the mode switch, and (6) the intensity control. Depending on the type of stimulation device, there may be a number of other switches including: a polarity switch, a pulse width control, and so forth. Note the wide variety of terms that are used to represent each of the control features on different machines. Even the same manufacturer of different machines may not use the same term to represent the intensity or frequency control. On one machine, the manufacturer may label the intensity control the *power* switch, on another machine it may be labeled *intensity* or *output*.

Note the particular electrode arrangement that is used with the stimulation device. The following are common: (1) two to four channels usually are seen with AC sine wave stimulators (each of the channels is separate and the therapist may use any number of channels for the stimulation procedure), (2) two channels are used with an interferential current stimulator, and (3) one electrode with two leads plus a separate dispersive or ground electrode usually is seen with a high-voltage stimulator. Note whether the stimulation device has a probe electrode and whether it has an ultrasound unit contained in the device.

Next, move to a different electrical stimulation device. Identify the type of electrical stimulator and identify the various parts as before. Although many of the stimulators have control knobs, some of them may have computerized panels and controls. It should be pointed out that regardless of the type of controls or the complexity of the machine, electrical current has the same effect on the patient. It might be helpful to draw the faceplate of each of the stimulators on a piece of paper and label the various parts.

Electrical Stimulation Laboratory Exercise #2: Understanding Current Parameters

Step 1. Position yourself at any of the electrical stimulation devices and identify the features as you did in Lab exercise #1. Connect the electrodes from one channel over the extensor muscles of your forearm. Place one of the electrodes on the skin approximately 2 inches distal to the elbow and the second electrode midway between the elbow and the wrist. Note that if you are using a high-voltage stimulator, you also need a third electrode, the dispersive or ground electrode. If you wish to use the large 8 inch by 10 inch pad that is provided, place it under the thigh (be sure to use a moist sponge with this electrode). You may substitute a smaller pad for the large dispersive pad and it can be placed on the upper arm, the thigh, or the lower back.

Step 2. Before proceeding, make sure that each of the intensity controls is set at zero. If it is a rotating knob, the zero position will be fully counterclockwise. Although most stimulation devices have built-in safety switches to minimize the risk of alarming the patient, resetting the equipment each time is a good habit to develop. Some machines have a toggle that is built into the intensity switch. If this is the case, the toggle must be engaged to start the machine. Turn on the power to the machine. Many of the newer devices are designed to run self-checks each time they are powered up and you may notice a few blinking lights at this stage. Once the machine is active, set the controls at the following:

frequency	100 Hz
mode	continuous
time	15 minutes

Step 3. Doublecheck your electrodes to make sure they are connected to both the machine and your arm. Now, start the timer by pressing the start button. Slowly begin to raise the intensity of the channel that is connected to your arm. As you begin to raise the current intensity notice that there is no sensation at first. However, as current intensity is raised, it will reach sufficient intensity to depolarize the large superficial sensory nerves. At this point, a sensation of mild "pins and needles" will be felt. This is the sensory level stimulus or SLS that was described earlier in the text. Once the pins and needles sensation is achieved, stop raising the current for a minute or so and notice what happens to the sensation. It will typically decrease, perhaps even disappear. This occurs because the body has adapted or accommodated to the sensation. This adaptation may or may not be helpful and we will look at different ways of increasing and decreasing adaptation in the next exercise.

Note: When using electrical stimulation for patient care, it is helpful to inform patients that this "pins and needles" sensation will occur. Patients are not likely to be concerned about this sensation because most have previously experienced a similar feeling.

Step 4. After allowing the body to adapt to the current intensity level, begin to slowly raise the current again. Notice that the pins and needles feeling returns and increases in intensity. If the sensation becomes uncomfortable, stop increasing the current for a few seconds and allow the body to adapt again. Usually, after a short time, it is acceptable to begin to raise the current again. As the current intensity continues to rise, the sensation will become stronger and stronger. This is because the increased current depolarizes more and more sensory fibers. At a certain point, usually about 15 to 20 mA, the current becomes sufficiently strong to depolarize some of the motor nerves. At this point, a muscle contraction should occur. It may be necessary to modify the electrode position slightly to achieve a muscle contraction. If the stimulation becomes too uncomfortable before a contraction is achieved, turn the current intensity back to zero, move the electrodes, and slowly increase the current intensity as before.

Step 5. With the current parameters placed at the above settings, you should be experiencing a constant or tetanizing muscle contraction of the wrist. The next step is to modify the frequency setting and observe what happens to the muscle contraction. Identify the frequency control knob and slowly decrease the frequency of the current. Note that as you decrease the frequency of the stimulation, the sensation diminishes slightly. This is because the current is not present as often. If the current becomes too weak to continue the muscle contraction, it may be necessary to gradually increase the current intensity again. Continue to decrease the current frequency until you reach 20 Hz. At this point, you should still be experiencing a steady, tetanizing contraction of the wrist. Slowly decrease the frequency and notice the point at which the contraction changes. Rather than continuing a steady contraction, the muscle will begin to twitch. This is a nontetanized contraction and the rate of twitch is controlled by the frequency. As the frequency is reduced to less than 10 Hz, the twitches should become more noticeable. Slowly increase the current frequency once again and notice the point at which tetany occurs.

Step 6. Turn the machine off and start again. In this section of the laboratory exercise, we will look at the difference between a continuous and an interrupted mode. Place the controls at the settings used in Step 2 (*i.e.*, 100 Hz continuous mode for 15 minutes). Start the machine and raise the current to the gentle sensory level as before. Allow the current to remain at this level for a minute or so and notice the adaptation that occurs.

Next, identify the mode control. Set the ON time at 5 seconds and the OFF time at 5 seconds. Now change the mode from a continuous setting to a surged or interrupted setting. Notice that now the current is delivered for a short period of time and then disappears completely. When the current returns, it will typically increase gradually over a short period, usually 1 second. This is referred to as the "ramp" and is used to improve patient comfort. Allow the current to remain at this sensory level on the interrupted mode for several minutes and notice the difference in sensation compared with the continuous mode. One of the advantages of the interrupted mode is the increased level of patient awareness.

Step 7. Turn the machine off and set the following parameters: 40 Hz, interrupted mode (5 seconds ON and 5 seconds OFF), and 15 minutes. Start the stimulator and gradually raise the current to produce a muscle contraction (motor level). Observe that the muscle alternately contracts and relaxes.

Note: It is important to be careful to raise the current only during the time that the current is ON. If you continue to raise current during the OFF time, it might become too intense and shock the patient when it returns. It is somewhat cumbersome to create the appropriate current intensity when using such a short ON time. To make it easier to set the current intensity at the desired level, it may be helpful to increase the ON time to 30 seconds, which allows adequate time to produce the desired muscle contraction. Once the current is sufficient to produce the contraction, reduce the ON time to 5 seconds.

At the conclusion of this laboratory exercise, you should understand the roles played by current intensity, current frequency, and current mode. Current intensity determines what type of nerves respond (*i.e.*, sensory, motor, or noxious). For example, there must be enough current present to depolarize a motor nerve in order to elicit a muscle contraction. Current frequency, in contrast, determines how the nerve responds. As you have seen, once a muscle contraction occurs (current intensity), the type of contraction can be modified by using the frequency control. Variations in current mode are used to modify patient adaptation to the stimulus and to modify the contraction. Most of the treatment protocols are a combination of current intensity, frequency, and mode. By understanding the function of each of these current parameters, the student will have gained a significant appreciation for the treatment protocols.

Electrical Stimulation Laboratory Exercise #3— Electrode Placement Techniques

Pain Control: HiTENS—Acute Pain in the Lower Back

Step 1. Select a stimulator that uses an alternating, sinusoidal current for this procedure. Position your lab partner in a prone position on the therapy table and expose the skin of the lower back. Using two channels and four electrodes, place the electrodes on the skin over the lower back. The electrodes should be placed in either of the following ways: (1) both electrodes from channel 1 placed on the left side of the spine and both electrodes from channel 2 placed on the right side, (2) the electrodes can be crossed in an interferential-like arrangement. In this configuration, the electrodes from channel 1 can be placed at the 10 o'clock and 4 o'clock positions, while the electrodes from channel 2 can be placed at the 2 o'clock and 8 o'clock positions.

Step 2. Next, set the parameters as follows: (1) frequency—80 to 150 Hz, (2) mode—continuous, (3) time—15 minutes. Doublecheck to make sure the patient is comfortable. Start the stimulator and slowly raise the current intensity until your lab partner begins to feel a slight tingling sensation. Note that this sensation fades slightly over the first few minutes and it may be necessary to increase the intensity. If the patient experiences any muscle contractions, reduce the intensity slightly.

Pain Control: LoTENS - Chronic Lower Back Pain with Sciatica

Step 1. Select a high-voltage stimulator for this procedure. Position your lab partner in a prone position on the therapy table and expose the skin of the lower back and the posterior thigh. Place the large 8 inch × 10 inch dispersive pad on the lower back. Place one of the active electrodes in the middle of the thigh at the gluteal crease. Place the second active electrode in the middle of the posterior thigh. It is helpful to use small active electrodes for this procedure.

Step 2. Next, set the parameters as follows: (1) frequency—1 to 5 Hz, (2) mode—continuous, (3) time—30 minutes. Doublecheck to make sure the patient is comfortable. Start the stimulator and slowly raise the current intensity until your lab partner begins to feel a tingling sensation. Gradually raise the current intensity until you begin to see muscle contractions of the buttocks and posterior thigh. Increase the current intensity to the maximal level that the patient will tolerate. This should be a strong motor level stimulus (MLS). Note the individual's reaction to the stimulus. It might be helpful to compare the response of your lab partner to other individuals. As stated, the response to any modality is quite varied. What one patient can tolerate, another cannot.

Pain Control: Conduction Block—Acute Pain in the Upper Back

Step 1. Select an interferential stimulator for this procedure. Position your lab partner in a prone position on the therapy table and expose the skin of the upper back. Using two channels and four electrodes, place the electrodes on the skin over the upper back. The electrodes should be crossed in an interferential-like arrangement. In this configuration, the electrodes from channel 1 can be placed at the 10 o'clock and 4 o'clock positions, while the electrodes from channel 2 can be placed at the 2 o'clock and 8 o'clock positions.

Step 2. Next, set the parameters as follows: (1) frequency—5000 Hz, (2) mode—continuous, (3) time—15 minutes. Doublecheck to make sure the patient is comfortable. Start the stimulator and slowly raise the current intensity until your lab partner begins to feel a slight tingling sensation. Note that this sensation fades slightly over the first few minutes and it may be necessary to increase the intensity. If the patient experiences any muscle contractions, reduce the intensity slightly.

Brief, Intense TENS: Myofascial Trigger Points in the Upper Back

Step 1. Identify a myofascial trigger point in the upper trapezius or levator scapulae muscle. Evaluate the length of the muscle and compare it to the one on the opposite side.

Step 2. Select a high-voltage stimulator with a probe electrode for this procedure. Position your lab partner in a seated position on the therapy table and expose the skin of the upper back. Because of the necessary high intensity used with this protocol, it is helpful to use the large 8 inch × 10 inch dispersive pad. Place the dispersive electrode under the patient's thigh. Place some coupling gel in the area over the trigger point and place the probe electrode directly on the myofascial trigger point.

Step 3. Set the parameters as follows: (1) frequency -100 Hz, (2) mode—probe, (3) time—15 minutes. Doublecheck to make sure the patient is comfortable. Start the stimulator and slowly raise the current intensity until your lab partner begins to feel a slight tingling sensation. Continue to raise the current intensity until you see a muscle contraction. Note that you may need to move the probe electrode slightly to maximize the muscle contraction. Raise the intensity until you achieve a strong muscle contraction and keep the probe in contact for 30 seconds.

Step 4. Stop the stimulation by removing the probe electrode. Reduce the intensity of the current to zero and place the probe on the therapy table. Stretch the muscle containing the myofascial trigger point that you have been treating.

Step 5. Replace the probe electrode on the TP and repeat the procedure. It is important to make sure that the current is reduced before replacing the probe on the patient. After several repetitions of the stimulation and stretch procedure, re-evaluate the muscle length and note any changes.

Combination Ultrasound—Electrical Stimulation: Myofascial Trigger Points in the Upper Back

Step 1. Identify a myofascial trigger point in the upper trapezius or levator scapulae muscle. Evaluate the length of the muscle and compare to the opposite side.

Step 2. Select a high-voltage stimulator with a combination ultrasound for this procedure. Position your lab partner in a seated position on the therapy table and expose the skin of the upper back. Place the large dispersive electrode under the patient's thigh. Place some coupling gel in the area over the trigger point and place the ultrasound head directly on the myofascial trigger point.

Step 3. Set the electrical stimulation parameters as follows: (1) frequency—100 Hz, (2) mode—combination, (3) time—8 minutes. Doublecheck to make sure the patient is comfortable. Start the stimulator and slowly raise the current intensity until your lab partner begins to feel a slight tingling sensation. Continue to raise the current intensity until you see a muscle contraction. Note that you may need to move the ultrasound head slightly to maximize the muscle contraction. Raise the intensity until you achieve a strong muscle contraction and ultrasound head in contact.

Step 4. Next, set the ultrasound parameters. The duty cycle should be set on 100% and the intensity at 1.5 w/cm^2. Once you begin to raise the intensity of the ultrasound it is important that you maintain constant motion of the ultrasound head.

Step 5. At the completion of the treatment, remove the ultrasound head and wipe the coupling gel off the patient. Next, stretch the muscle while it is warm and pliable. Re-evaluate the muscle length and note any changes.

Muscle Spasms in the Lower Back

Step 1. Select a stimulator that uses an alternating, sinusoidal current for this procedure. Position your lab partner in a prone position on the therapy table and expose the skin of the lower back. Using two channels and four electrodes, place the electrodes on the skin over the lower back. The electrodes should be placed in either of the following ways: (1) both electrodes from channel 1 placed on the left side of the spine and both electrodes from channel 2 placed on the right side, and (2) the electrodes can be crossed in an interferential-like arrangement. In this configuration, the electrodes from channel 1 may be placed at the 10 o'clock and 4 o'clock positions, while the electrodes from channel 2 may be placed at the 2 o'clock and 8 o'clock positions.

Step 2. Next, set the parameters as follows: (1) frequency—80 to 150 Hz, (2) mode—continuous, (3) time—15 minutes. Doublecheck to make sure the patient is comfortable. Start the stimulator and slowly raise the current intensity until your lab partner begins to feel a slight tingling sensation. Continue to raise the current intensity until a muscle contraction is seen. Because muscle contractions in the lower back may be difficult to see, it may be necessary to palpate the muscle to identify the point at which a contraction occurs.

Step 3. Reduce the current intensity to zero and change the treatment mode setting to surged. Place the ON time at 30 seconds and the OFF time at 5 seconds. Start the stimulator and, while the current is ON, raise the intensity to a motor level, as before. When a muscle contraction is achieved, reduce the ON time to 5 seconds. Note any difference in the patient's perception of the two methods.

Range of Motion of the Ankle

Step 1. Select a stimulator that uses an alternating, sinusoidal current for this procedure. Position your lab partner in a supine position on the therapy table and expose the skin of the leg and ankle. It is helpful to place a small pillow under the leg for this procedure. Using two channels and four electrodes, place the electrodes from channel 1 on the motor points of the anterior shin. The electrodes from channel 2 should be placed on the motor points of the gastrocnemius muscle.

Step 2. Set the parameters as follows: (1) frequency—20 to 50 Hz, (2) mode—reciprocating, (3) time—15 minutes. Doublecheck to make sure the patient is comfortable. Start the stimulator and begin to raise the current intensity. Note that the current will switch back and forth from channel 1 to channel 2. This switching of the current will occur at whatever interval is set on the stimulator. If possible, set the ON time for each current at 30 seconds, which will allow adequate time to set the desired current intensity before the current switches. Once the current is at a motor level on each channel, reduce the ON time to 5 seconds.

Step 3. If the desired muscle contraction does not occur, reduce the current intensity and move the electrodes slightly. Start the current and gradually raise the intensity as before. It may be necessary to move the electrodes several times to achieve the desired level of contraction.

Tissue Healing

Step 1. Select an interferential current stimulator for this procedure. Position your lab partner in a supine position on the therapy table and expose the knee. It is helpful to place a small pillow under the leg for this procedure. The electrodes should be crossed in an interferential-like arrangement. In this configuration, the electrodes from channel 1 may be placed at the 10 o'clock and 4 o'clock positions, while the electrodes from channel 2 may be placed at the 2 o'clock and 8 o'clock positions.

Step 2. Set the parameters as follows: (1) frequency—1 to 15 Hz, (2) mode—quadpolar, (3) time—15 minutes. Doublecheck to make sure the patient is comfortable. Start the stimulator and begin to raise the current intensity until a rapid twitching contraction begins to occur in the muscles around the knee.

Step 3. If the desired muscle contraction does not occur, reduce the current intensity and move the electrodes slightly. Start the current and gradually raise the intensity as before. It may be necessary to move the electrodes several times to achieve the desired level of contraction.

Traction

Lumbar Traction: Low Back Pain (Orthion Table)

Step 1. Place the upper trunk portion of the traction harness on the traction table and secure it to the table. Place the lumbar harness around your lab partner. The top of the harness should be located at the superior portion of the crest of the ilium.

Step 2. Place your lab partner in a supine position on the traction table. It is helpful to place a cushion or pillow under the knees. Wrap the upper traction harness around the patient's chest and secure the straps. The harness should be placed in such a way that it may be securely fastened to the rib cage, not the abdomen.

Step 3. Attach the belt that extends from the lower harness to the upper hole in the lumbar post. Tighten all of the straps and check to see that the patient is comfortable.

Step 4. Set the parameters of the traction table at: (1) 50 pounds, (2) static traction, and (3) 20 minutes. Provide the hand-held cut-off switch to the patient.

Step 5. Begin the traction treatment and note that the traction force is gradually increased over a period of several minutes. Note where in the spine the traction force is greatest.

Step 6. Stop the traction treatment. Reposition the lower belt to the middle hole on the lumbar post and repeat Step 5. Note where the traction force is greatest. Repeat once again with the belt attached to the lower hole.

Step 7. Stop the traction treatment. Change the traction parameters to (1) 70 pounds hold force, (2) 40 pounds rest force, (3) 30 seconds hold time, (4) 10 seconds rest time, and (5) 20 minutes. Begin the traction procedure again and note any difference in the sensation that the patient experiences.

Cervical Traction: Neck Pain (Orthion Table)

Step 1. Place the cervical traction harness on the traction table and secure it to the table.

Step 2. Place your lab partner in a supine position on the traction table. It is helpful to place a cushion or pillow under the knees. Place the cervical traction harness around the patient's head. The harness should be placed in such a way that it rests against the occiput. Position the chin strap and secure it to the head harness.

Step 3. Attach the belt that extends from the traction harness to the upper hole in the cervical post. Tighten all of the straps and check to see that the patient is comfortable.

Step 4. Set the parameters of the traction table at: (1) 10 pounds, (2) static traction, and (3) 20 minutes. Provide the hand-held cut-off switch to the patient.

Step 5. Begin the traction treatment and note that the traction force is gradually increased over a period of several minutes. Note where in the spine the traction force is greatest.

Step 6. Stop the traction treatment. Reposition the traction harness to: the middle hole on the cervical post and repeat Step 5. Note where the traction force is greatest. Repeat once again with the belt attached to the lower hole.

Step 7. Stop the traction treatment. Change the traction parameters to (1) 20 pounds hold force, (2) 10 pounds rest force, (3) 30 seconds hold time, (4) 10 seconds rest time, and (5) 20 minutes. Begin the traction procedure again and note any difference in the sensation that the patient experiences.

Cervical Traction: Over-the-Door Harness

Step 1. Place the over-the-door apparatus over the top of a door. Position a chair under the apparatus in such a way that the chair faces the door. Place 1 gallon of water (approximately 8 pounds) in the weight bag.

Step 2. Attach the cervical halter to the patient.

Step 3. Sit the patient in the chair, facing the door. Attach the halter to: the over-the-door apparatus. Note where the traction force is felt.

Step 4. Change the position of the patient by moving the chair closer and then farther away from the door and note any differences in the location of the traction force experienced by the patient.

Step 5. Turn the chair around so the patient is seated with his or her back to the door. Change the position of the chair several times, as before, and note any differences in the location of the traction forces.

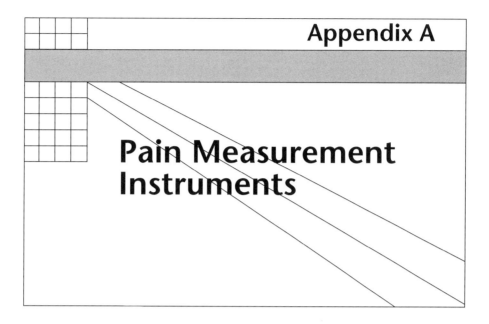

Appendix A

Pain Measurement Instruments

How and When to Use

1. At initial evaluation and prior to initiating any treatment, the following pain measurement tools can be used:
   - Visual Analog Scale
   - pain drawing
   - pain questionnaire (select an appropriate pain questionnaire from those provided)

2. During the course of treatment, it may be helpful periodically to assess the level of pain and disability to measure improvement. The following assessment strategy is suggested:
   - Visual Analog Scale: perform once weekly while the patient remains in pain.

Note: It is acceptable to use a verbal scale by simply asking the patient to rate the pain on a scale of 0 to 10. Be sure to note the response in the patient's daily record.

   - pain drawing: it is helpful to have the patient redo the pain drawing at the time of any formal re-evaluation or re-examination. This can be as often as every 2 weeks but should probably be done at least once monthly.
   - pain questionnaire: it may be helpful to use this tool on a monthly basis and at the time the patient is released from care.

Visual Analog Scale: Pain Drawing

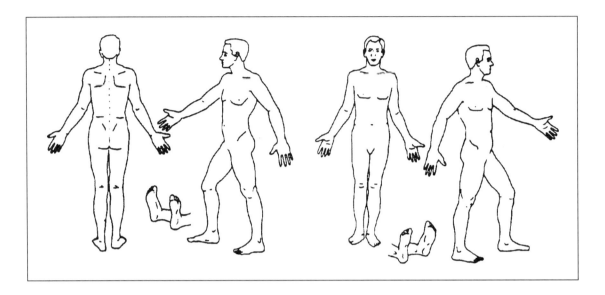

Numbness	= = = =	Burning	x x x x
Pins and needles	o o o o	Stabbing	/ / / /
Aching	a a a a		

Instructions for Scoring

Writing anywhere on the drawing	1
No physiologic pain pattern	1
No physiologic sensory change	1
More than one type of pain	1
Both upper and lower areas of the body involved	1
Markings outside the body	1
Unspecified symbols	1

Score: 1 = Normal   5 or more = Very bad

Pain Questionnaires: Which to Use

1. Neck pain
   a. Neck Pain Disability Questionnaire
2. Back pain
   a. Oswestry Low Back Pain Disability Questionnaire
   b. Roland Morris Low Back Pain Disability Questionnaire
3. Other pain
   a. McGill Pain Questionnaire

Neck Pain Disability Index

How to Use

This questionnaire has been designed to give the doctor information as to how your neck pain has affected your ability to manage in everyday life. Please answer every section and mark in each section only the ONE box that applies to you. We realize you may consider that two of the statements in any one section relate to you, but please just mark the box which most closely describes your problem.

Section 1: Pain Intensity

- ☐ I have no pain at the moment.
- ☐ The pain is very mild at the moment.
- ☐ The pain is moderate at the moment.
- ☐ The pain is fairly severe at the moment.
- ☐ The pain is very severe at the moment.
- ☐ The pain is the worst imaginable at the moment.

Section 2: Personal Care (washing, dressing, and so forth)

- ☐ I can look after myself normally without experiencing extra pain.
- ☐ I can look after myself normally but it causes extra pain.
- ☐ It is painful to look after myself and I am slow and careful.
- ☐ I need some help but manage most of my personal care.
- ☐ I need help every day in most aspects of self-care.
- ☐ I do not get dressed, I wash with difficulty, and I stay in bed.

Section 3: Lifting

- ☐ I can lift heavy weights without extra pain.
- ☐ I can lift heavy weights but it gives extra pain.
- ☐ Pain prevents me from lifting heavy weights off the floor, but I can manage if they are conveniently positioned, for example on a table.
- ☐ Pain prevents me from lifting heavy weights, but I can manage light to medium weights if they are conveniently positioned.
- ☐ I can lift very light weights.
- ☐ I cannot lift or carry anything at all.

Section 4: Reading

- ☐ I can read as much as I want to with no pain in my neck.
- ☐ I can read as much as I want to with slight pain in my neck.

☐ I can read as much as I want to with moderate pain in my neck.

☐ I cannot read as much as I want because of moderate pain in my neck.

☐ I can hardly read at all because of severe pain in my neck.

☐ I cannot read at all.

Section 5: Headaches

☐ I have no headaches at all.

☐ I have slight headaches that come infrequently.

☐ I have moderate headaches that come infrequently.

☐ I have moderate headaches that come frequently.

☐ I have severe headaches that come frequently.

☐ I have headaches almost all of the time.

Section 6: Concentration

☐ I can concentrate fully when I want to with no difficulty.

☐ I can concentrate fully when I want to with slight difficulty.

☐ I have a fair degree of difficulty in concentrating when I want to.

☐ I have a lot of difficulty in concentrating when I want to.

☐ I have a great deal of difficulty in concentrating when I want to.

☐ I cannot concentrate at all.

Section 7: Work

☐ I can do as much work as I want to.

☐ I can only do my usual work, but no more.

☐ I can do most of my usual work, but no more.

☐ I cannot do my usual work.

☐ I can hardly do any work at all.

☐ I cannot do any work at all.

Section 8: Driving

☐ I can drive my car without any neck pain.

☐ I can drive my car as long as I want with slight pain in my neck.

☐ I can drive my car as long as I want with moderate pain in my neck.

☐ I cannot drive my car as long as I want because of moderate pain in my neck.

☐ I can hardly drive at all because of severe pain in my neck.

☐ I cannot drive my car at all.

Section 9: Sleeping

☐ I have no trouble sleeping.

☐ My sleep is slightly disturbed (less than 1 hour sleepless).

☐ My sleep is mildly disturbed (1 to 2 hours sleepless).

☐ My sleep is moderately disturbed (2 to 3 hours sleepless).

☐ My sleep is greatly disturbed (3 to 5 hours sleepless).

☐ My sleep is completely disturbed (5 to 7 hours sleepless).

Section 10: Recreation

☐ I am able to engage in all my recreation activities with no neck pain at all.

☐ I am able to engage in all my recreation activities with some pain in my neck.

☐ I am able to engage in most, but not all, of my usual recreation activities because of pain in my neck.

☐ I am able to engage in only a few of my usual recreation activities because of pain in my neck.

☐ I can hardly do any recreation activities because of pain in my neck.

☐ I cannot do any recreation activities at all.

Instructions on Scoring

For each section, scores fall on a 0 to 5 scale, with the higher values representing greater disability. The sum of the 10 scores is expressed as a percentage of the maximal score. If a patient fails to complete a section, the percentage is adjusted accordingly.

0% to 10%	=	no disability
11% to 30%	=	minimal (mild) disability
31% to 50%	=	moderate disability
51% to 70%	=	severe disability
>70%	=	completely disabled by pain in several areas of life

Oswestry Pain Questionnaire

How to Use

This questionnaire is designed to help us understand how much your low back pain has affected your ability to manage your everyday activities. Please answer each section by circling the ONE CHOICE that most applies to you. We realize that you may feel that more than one statement may relate to you, but please, just circle the ONE choice that most closely describes your problem right now.

Section 1: Pain Intensity

☐ The pain comes and goes and is very mild.

☐ The pain is mild and does not vary much.

☐ The pain comes and goes and is moderate.

☐ The pain is moderate and does not vary much.

☐ The pain comes and goes and is severe.

☐ The pain is severe and does not vary much.

Section 2: Personal Care

☐ I do not have to change my way of washing or dressing to avoid pain.

☐ I do not normally change my way of washing or dressing even though it causes some pain.

☐ Washing and dressing increases the pain but I manage not to change my way of doing so.

☐ Washing and dressing increases the pain and I find it necessary to change my way of doing so.

☐ Because of the pain I am unable to do some washing and dressing without help.

☐ Because of the pain I am unable to do any washing and dressing without help.

Section 3: Lifting

☐ I can lift heavy weights without extra pain.

☐ I can lift heavy weights but it causes extra pain.

☐ Pain prevents me from lifting heavy weights off the floor.

☐ Pain prevents me from lifting heavy weights off the floor, but I can manage if they are conveniently positioned, for example, on a table.

☐ Pain prevents me from lifting heavy weights, but I can manage light to medium weights if they are conveniently positioned.

☐ I can only lift very light weights at the most.

Section 4: Walking

☐ I have no pain on walking.

☐ I have some pain on walking but it does not increase with distance.

☐ I cannot walk more than one half mile without increasing pain.

☐ I cannot walk more than one quarter mile without increasing pain.

☐ I cannot walk at all without increasing pain.

Section 5: Sitting

☐ I can sit in any chair as long as I like.

☐ I can sit only in my favorite chair as long as I like.

☐ Pain prevents me from sitting more than 1 hour.

☐ Pain prevents me from sitting more than one half hour.

☐ Pain prevents me from sitting more than 10 minutes.

☐ I avoid sitting because it increases pain straight away.

Section 6: Standing

☐ I can stand as long as I want without pain.

☐ I have some pain on standing but it does not increase with time.

☐ I cannot stand for longer than 1 hour without increasing pain.

☐ I cannot stand for longer than one half hour without increasing pain.

☐ I cannot stand for longer than 10 minutes without increasing pain.

☐ I avoid standing because it increases the pain immediately.

Section 7: Sleeping

☐ I have no pain in bed.

☐ I have pain in bed but it does not prevent me from sleeping well.

☐ Because of pain, my normal night's sleep is reduced by one quarter.

☐ Because of pain, my normal night's sleep is reduced by one half.

☐ Because of pain, my normal night's sleep is reduced by three quarters.

☐ Pain prevents me from sleeping at all.

Section 8: Social Life

☐ My social life is normal and gives me no pain at all.

☐ My social life is normal but increases the degree of my pain.

☐ Pain has no significant effect on my social life apart from limiting my more energetic interests (*e.g.*, dancing).

☐ Pain has restricted my social life to my home.

☐ I have hardly any social life because of the pain.

Section 9: Traveling

☐ I get no pain while traveling.

☐ I get some pain while traveling, but none of my usual forms of travel make it any worse.

☐ I get extra pain while traveling, but it does not compel me to seek alternative forms of travel.

☐ I get extra pain while traveling, which compels me to seek alternative forms of travel.

☐ Pain restricts all forms of travel.

☐ Pain prevents all forms of travel except that done lying down.

Section 10: Changing Degree of Pain

☐ My pain is rapidly getting better.

☐ My pain fluctuates but overall is definitely getting better.

☐ My pain seems to be getting better but improvement is slow at present.

☐ My pain is getting neither better nor worse.

☐ My pain is gradually worsening.

☐ My pain is rapidly worsening.

Instructions on Scoring

For each section, scores fall on a scale from 0 to 5, with the higher values representing greater disability. Add the scores for all sections, divide by the total possible (50 points if all sections are completed; deduct 5 points from this for each uncompleted or missed section) and multiply by 100%.

Example:

$$\frac{15 \text{ (total points)}}{50 \text{ (total possible)}} \times \frac{100}{1} = 33.33\%$$

Disability Rating:

0% to 20%	=	minimal disability
21% to 40%	=	moderate disability
41% to 60%	=	severe disability
61% to 80%	=	crippling disability
81% to 100%	=	bedbound or exaggerating

Roland Morris Low Back Pain Disability Questionnaire

How to Use

When your back hurts, you may find it difficult to do some of the things you normally do. This list contains some sentences that people have used to describe themselves when they have back pain. When you read them, you may find that some stand out because they describe you *today*. When you read a sentence that describes yourself *today*, put a check mark in the box next to it. If the sentence does not describe you, then leave the space blank and go on to the next one. Remember, check only those sentences that you are sure describe you today.

- ☐ I stay at home most of the time because of my back.
- ☐ I change position frequently to try and get my back comfortable.
- ☐ I walk more slowly than usual because of my back.
- ☐ Because of my back, I am not doing any of the jobs that I usually do around the house.
- ☐ Because of my back, I use a handrail to get up stairs.
- ☐ Because of my back, I lie down to rest more often.
- ☐ Because of my back, I have to hold on to something to get out of an easy chair.
- ☐ Because of my back, I try to get other people to do things for me.
- ☐ I get dressed more slowly than usual because of my back.
- ☐ I stand up for only short periods of time because of my back.
- ☐ Because of my back, I try not to bend or kneel down.
- ☐ I find it difficult to get out of a chair because of my back.
- ☐ My back is painful almost all the time.
- ☐ I find it difficult to turn over in bed because of my back.
- ☐ My appetite is not very good because of my back.
- ☐ I have trouble putting on my socks (or stockings) because of the pain in my back.
- ☐ I walk only short distances because of my back pain.
- ☐ I sleep less well because of my back.
- ☐ Because of my back pain, I get dressed with help from someone else.
- ☐ I sit down for most of the day because of my back.
- ☐ I avoid heavy jobs around the house because of my back.
- ☐ Because of my back pain, I am more irritable and bad tempered with people than usual.
- ☐ Because of my back, I go upstairs more slowly than usual.
- ☐ I stay in bed most of the time because of my back.

Instructions on Scoring

Add the number of sentences that are checked by the patient. This should result in a score between 0 and 24. The patient is asked to put a mark next to each statement or leave it blank. If a word such as *sometimes* is written next to the sentence, this can be scored as a half point and added into the total.

On successive use, the Roland Morris Index will provide a percentage reduction in disability or improvement in function. This scale is more sensitive for patients in acute pain.

Assume a patient has a pretreatment score of 12. This is followed 2 weeks later by a score of 7, and 4 weeks later a score of 3. The overall improvement in function is 75%. This is calculated as follows:

$$\frac{9 \text{ (points of improvement during treatment)}}{12 \text{ (pretreatment score)}} \times \frac{100}{1} = 75\%$$

McGill Pain Questionnaire

How to Use

Look carefully at the 20 groups of words. If any word in any group applies to your pain, please circle that word—but do not circle more than *one word in any one group*—so you must choose the *most suitable word* in that group. In groups that do not apply to your pain, there is no need to circle *any* word—just leave them as they are.

Instructions on Use
Look carefully at the twenty groups of words. If any word in any group applies to your pain, please circle that word - but do not circle more than **one word in any given group** - so you must choose the **most suitable word** in that group. In groups that do not apply to your pain, there is no need to circle **any** word - just leave them as they are.

Group 1	Group 2	Group 3	Group 4	Group 5
Flickering Quivering Pulsing Throbbing Beating	Jumping Flashing Shooting	Pricking Boring Drilling Stabbing Lancinating	Sharp Gritting Lacerating	Pinching Pressing Gnawing Cramping Crushing
Group 6	Group 7	Group 8	Group 9	Group 10
Tugging Pulling Wrenching	Hot Burning Scalding Searing	Tingling Itching Smarting Stinging	Dull Sore Hurting Aching Heavy	Tender Taut Rasping Splitting
Group 11	Group 12	Group 13	Group 14	Group 15
Tiring Exhausting	Sickening Suffocating	Fearful Frightful Terrifying	Punishing Grueling Cruel Vicious Killing	Wretched Blinding
Group 16	Group 17	Group 18	Group 19	Group 20
Annoying Troublesome Miserable Intense Unbearable	Spreading Radiating Penetrating Piercing	Tight Numb Drawing Squeezing Tearing	Cool Cold Freezing	Nagging Nauseating Agonizing Dreadful Torturing

Instructions on Scoring

Patients are asked to circle not more than one word that best describes their pain in any of the 20 groups of words. The simplest scoring methods involve:

1. Total number of words circled
2. Intensity, measured by allotting score 1 to the first word in any group, 2 to the second, and so forth.

The first 10 groups of words are somatic or subjective. They are used to describe what the pain feels like to the patient. Groups 11 through 15 are affective and are used to describe the affect the pain has on the patient. Group 16 is considered to be evaluative and is used to describe the patient's evaluation of the pain. Groups 17 through 20 are miscellaneous and are used to further describe the patient's pain.

Note: One important part of pain evaluation is consideration of whether or not the description and quantification provided by the patient makes sense in terms of the type of problem the patient has, the mechanism of injury, and the examination findings.

Becker's Red Flags of Spinal Diagnosis

Becker's Red Flags of Spinal Diagnosis can be used to identify patients who have significant psychosocial issues that are included in their symptom picture. Although these red flags should not be considered as absolute indicators, they may be helpful when considered with other clinical tools.

1. Symptom distortion in the history:
   - vague or implausible history of injury
   - vague or inconsistent pain description
   - elaborate imagery to describe pain
   - pain rated 9 or more on a scale of 10
   - symptom proliferation
   - total body pain
   - episodes of collapse, inability to move or sudden numbness

2. Distortion in the physical examination:
   - discrepancy between observed versus tested motion
   - discrepancy between sitting versus recumbent straight leg raising (SLR)
   - low back pain on gentle cervical compression
   - tenderness on gentle palpation (jumping jack syndrome)
   - patient grabs or pushes examiner's hands away
   - symptoms worsen or proliferate despite treatment

3. Personal style:
   - emergency room visits by ambulance for pain medication
   - narcotic overuse or dependence
   - blames current life problems on physical condition
   - insists illness is purely somatic and unrelated to stress
   - "Pain has changed my entire life."
   - "I just want to get rid of the pain and get on with my life."
   - "I keep my feelings inside," or "I don't show my feelings."
   - histrionic presentation, often as a strange limp

4. Interpersonal relations:
   - blames mood (irritable, depressed) on physical condition
   - has family member phone for medication (passive dependency)
   - patient angry at employer and is generally irritable
   - denies psychosocial problems or blames them on pain
   - critical of previous doctors

- history of doctor shopping
- patient angers or frustrates doctor

5. Work:
  - states, "I've worked all my life" in asserting former independence
  - describes inappropriate activity curtailment
  - has "learned to accept" invalid status as a victim
  - setback as return to work date approaches
  - multiple return to work date extensions
  - "fears" will be unable ever to work again

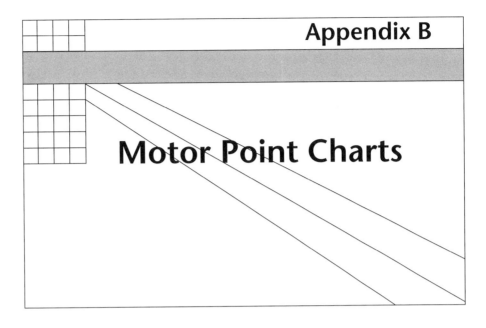

Appendix B

Motor Point Charts

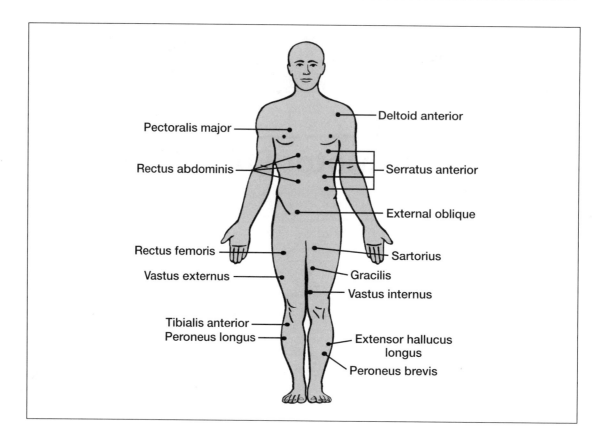

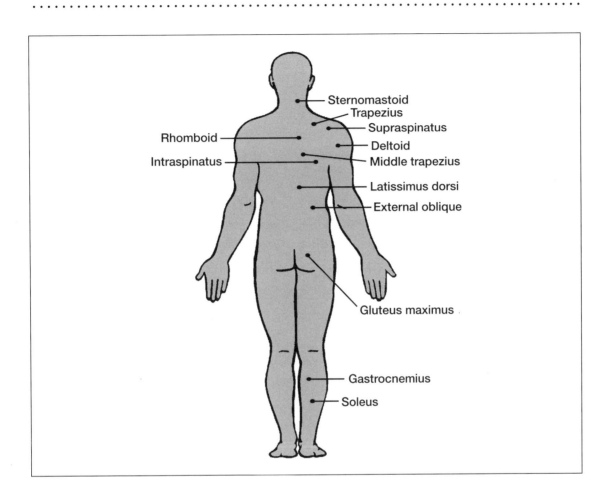

Sternomastoid
Trapezius
Supraspinatus
Rhomboid
Deltoid
Intraspinatus
Middle trapezius
Latissimus dorsi
External oblique
Gluteus maximus
Gastrocnemius
Soleus

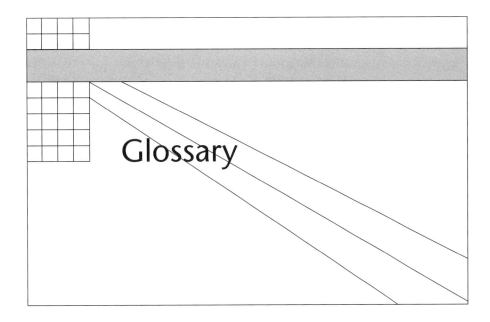

Glossary

A beta fibers large, rapidly conducting superficial sensory fibers; they provide the vehicle for TENS applications and the pain-gating mechanism

A delta fibers nociceptors that are mostly distributed throughout the superficial tissues of the body and in small numbers in the joints and muscles; they are sensitive to high- intensity mechanical stimuli

absolute positive, entire, complete, total

absolute contraindication a situation or condition that renders the use of a certain procedure or treatment inadvisable under any circumstances; no exceptions

absolute refractory period a brief time following membrane depolarization during which the membrane is incapable of depolarizing again, regardless of the strength of stimulus

absorption the taking up of fluids or other substances (energy) by the body

accommodation the adaptation of nerves to stimuli over time; accommodation is greater with a steady stimulus than with a variable stimulus

acoustic pertaining to sound or to the sense of hearing

acoustic spectrum the range of frequencies and wavelengths of sound waves; the form of energy used by therapeutic ultrasound

acoustic streaming a unidirectional movement in the tissues produced by the application of therapeutic ultrasound

ACTH adrenocorticotropic hormone (corticotropin); an adrenal cortex-stimulating hormone that is released by the anterior pituitary

actinic the ability of light waves to produce chemical effects

actinotherapy treatment of disease by rays of light

action potential a change in the electrical potential between the inside and outside of a cell, resulting in depolarization

active characterized by action; not passive

active electrode the electrode at which the greatest current density occurs

active range of motion that portion of the movement of a body part that a person can voluntarily create

active therapy those treatment procedures that involve some type of action on the part of the patient (*e.g.*, exercise)

acupressure a technique of using finger pressure over acupuncture points to decrease pain

acupuncture an ancient technique of health care that incorporates piercing the skin with needles in an attempt to restore a balance to the body's energy flow

acupuncturelike TENS treatment technique that involves electrical stimulation of acupuncture points to achieve pain relief; also referred to as LoTENS

acute having a short and relatively severe course

adhesions fibrous bands or structures by which parts abnormally stick together (adhere)

adjustment a change made to improve the current status

adsorption the attraction and holding of a gas or liquid on the surface of a substance

affective pertaining to a feeling or mental state

afferent the conduction of a nerve impulse from the periphery to the central nervous system (sensory)

afferent neuron nerves that convey information toward the central nervous system (sensory)

agonist a muscle or muscle group that is a prime mover and is ultimately responsible for a specific action

air space plate a capacitor type of electrode in which the plates are separated from the skin by an air space; used in shortwave diathermy

all-or-none response the depolarization of nerve or muscle membranes is always the same; however, once a particular current intensity is reached, depolarization occurs; greater intensities will not produce stronger responses

alternating current (AC) current that periodically changes its polarity or direction of flow

alternating mode an electrical stimulation parameter that involves the use of two electrical currents that are not active simultaneously; the current is directed to one channel, then to the other in an alternating manner; also referred to as a reciprocating mode

ampere a unit of measure that indicates the rate at which electrical current is flowing

amplifier an apparatus for increasing the volume or intensity of a sound or an electrical current

amplitude the intensity, as in the intensity of current flow

analgesia the loss of sensibility to pain

anaphoresis the transmission of positively charged ions into tissues by an electrical current

ancillary assisting in the achievement of a result; not primary

anesthesia the loss of sensation

angstrom an international unit used in measuring the wavelength of light

anion an ion carrying a negative charge and attracted to a positive pole

anode the positive pole of an electrical source

annulus fibrosus that part of the intervertebral disc consisting of interlacing cross fibers of fibroelastic tissue that are attached to adjacent vertebral bodies

anoxia a reduction of oxygen in the tissues

applicator the electrode used to transfer energy in microwave diathermy

Arndt-Schultz Principle for a reaction to occur in the body, the amount of energy absorbed must be sufficient to stimulate the absorbing tissues; weak stimuli increase physiologic activity and very strong stimuli inhibit or abolish activity

articular dealing with two or more bones joining together to form a joint

articular cartilage the smooth cartilage layer that lines the surface of synovial joints

ascending pathway a nerve pathway or spinal tract that has an upward course

assessment the process of evaluation

asymmetric not symmetric; dissimilar in corresponding body parts or organs on opposite sides of the body

attenuation the act of thinning or weakening; a decrease in energy due to either absorption or scattering of ultrasound waves

atonic without tone

autonomic self-controlling; functioning independently

autonomic nervous system that portion of the nervous system that functions without voluntary control

autotraction a specific form of traction involving a device that the patient is able to control

average current the average amount of current that is delivered during a stimulation; the result of an interaction between the peak current and the pulse width

avulsion a fracture in which a small piece of bone is torn away from its attachment by a tendon or ligament

beta-endorphin a neurohormone that is similar in structure to morphine and has similar analgesic properties

beta-lipotropin a pituitary hormone that is a precursor to beta-endorphin

biphasic current an alternating electrical current in which the direction of flow continually reverses

bipolar referring to the two poles used in electrotherapy

black light lamp an apparatus that produces Wood's rays to detect ultra-violet-fluorescent materials (*e.g.*, ringworm)

bradykinin a potent vasodilator that is released in injured tissue as part of the inflammatory process

brief, intense TENS a form of electrical stimulation with a short stimulus at a strong motor level intensity; a form of counterirritant

bursa a sac or saclike cavity filled with a viscid fluid and situated at places in the tissues at which friction would otherwise develop

bursts a combined set of three or more electrical pulses; also referred to as packets or envelopes

burst TENS a current modulation that uses a high frequency current that is divided into a series of bursts or packets

cable electrodes an inductance type of electrode in which the electrodes are coiled around the body part; used in shortwave diathermy

calcific bursitis hardening of the bursal sack with deposition of calcium

calcification hardening of tissue resulting from deposition of bone salts

capacitance a property of electric nonconductors that permits the storage of energy

capacitor a device consisting of conducting coils separated by thin layers of dielectric (*e.g.*, air) used in shortwave diathermy

cardiovascular pertaining to the heart and blood vessels

carpal tunnel the osteofibrous passage for the passage of the median nerve and the flexor tendons of the wrist

carpal tunnel syndrome a condition involving inflammation of the carpal tunnel; usually accompanied by irritation and pressure on the median nerve

cartilage a specialized form of connective tissue

cataphoresis the process of driving negative ions into tissues by using an electric current

cathode a negatively charged electrode in a direct current system

causalgia an extreme burning pain that represents a reflex vasomotor dystrophy

cavitation the mechanical vibration of small gas bubbles in the blood or body fluids that results in the formation of cavities

central biasing a theory of pain modulation

chilblains a localized erythema on the fingers produced by exposure to cold, damp weather

chronaxie the time necessary to cause depolarization, given a current of twice the rheobase intensity

chronic persisting over a long period of time

chronic condition a condition that has been present for approximately 6 to 7 weeks and is not showing signs of improvement

chronic obstructive pulmonary disease (COPD) a degenerative condition affecting the vascular, lymphatic, and pulmonary systems

chronic pain pain that has been present for at least 6 months

circuit the path of current from a generating source through the various components and back to the source

claudication a cramping pain due to ischemia

Cobb's angle a method of measuring scoliosis in which a line is drawn through the upper border of the cephalad vertebra that tilts to the concavity and then at the inferior border of the caudad vertebra that tilts most to the convexity; the angle is measured at the intersection of these two lines

collagen the main supportive protein of skin, tendon, bone, cartilage, and connective tissue

complement system a chemical system in the blood that aids in the destruction of pathogenic bacteria and materials

compliance the act of complying, yielding, or acting in accord

complicated injury an injury that involves trauma to different tissues and systems (*e.g.*, a bone fracture that also pierces the skin)

concentric a type of muscle contraction that shortens the muscle; used to accelerate or create motion

condenser electrodes an electrical current conducted back and forth between two electrodes; deep heating occurs between the electrodes

conductance the ease with which a current flows along a conducting medium

conduction heat loss or gain through direct contact (*e.g.,* hydrocollator packs and ice bags)

conduction block a mechanism of pain relief using various forms of high-frequency stimulation

congestion the presence of an abnormal amount of fluid in the vessels as a result of either an increase in blood or lymph flow or obstructed vascular or lymphatic return

connective tissue the fibrous tissue that pervades the entire body and serves to unite and support the various parts

constant current direct (galvanic) current; continuous nonpulsed current

continuous current an uninterrupted electrical current; may refer to either a pulsed or nonpulsed (galvanic) current

continuous passive movement (CPM) a mechanical device that is used to improve healing in the synovial joints

continuous traction a form of traction that involves the application of small amounts of weights for long periods of time

contraindication special symptoms or circumstances that render the use of a remedy or treatment procedure inadvisable

contrast bath alternating applications of hot (106°F) and cold (50°F) treatments to stimulate superficial vascular flow

contrast therapy alternating applications of heat and cold

convection heat loss or gain through the movement of air or water across the skin (*e.g.,* whirlpool or fluidotherapy)

conversion the process of changing one form of energy into another form (*e.g.,* electrical energy into ultrasound)

cosine law optimal radiation occurs when the source of radiation is at right angles to the area being radiated

coulomb an indication of the number of electrons flowing in a current

counterirritation a theory of pain modulation based on the idea that "pain inhibits pain"

coupling agent a substance used as a medium for the transfer of ultrasound waves (*e.g.,* water or gel)

cps an abbreviation for cycles per second; synonymous with hertz; a measure of frequency

cross friction massage a therapeutic massage technique that incorporates small circular movements that penetrate into the depth of a muscle to break fibrous tissue adhesions within a tendon, muscle or ligament

cryesthesia abnormal sensitivity to cold

cryanesthesia anesthesia produced by the application of cold

cryokinetics the combined use of cold and exercise in the treatment of musculoskeletal problems

cryotherapy the use of cold in the treatment of pathology and/or disease

crystal the part of the ultrasound head that vibrates and changes shape resulting in the emission of ultrasonic waves

current the flow of electrons

current density amount of current flow per cubic area

cycle one period of alternating current

decay time the time required for a waveform to go from peak amplitude to zero volts

deconditioning syndrome a condition involving a series of changes including weight gain, loss of muscle strength and endurance, and general atrophy; usually accompanies long periods of inactivity

degenerative joint disease (DJD) a condition involving deterioration in a synovial joint

depolarization the process of neutralizing the cell membranes resting potential

dermatome the topographic area of skin that is supplied by afferent cutaneous fibers from a single posterior spinal nerve

descending control system that portion of the neurologic system that extends downward and exerts control

descriptor pertaining to description or characterization

desiccation the process of drying out, or dehydrating

desquamation the shedding of epithelial tissues, especially of the skin

diagnosis the art of distinguishing one form of disease from another

diagnostic ultrasound a form of ultrasound that is used for diagnostic purposes

diapulse pulsed shortwave diathermy

diathermy the application of high-frequency electromagnetic energy to generate heat in the deeper body tissues

dielectric a nonconductor of direct electric current; an insulator between two electrically charged plates

diffuse not definitely limited or localized

diffusion the transfer of a substance from an area of greater to an area of lesser concentration

digital pressure pressure exerted by the fingers; often used for the treatment of acupuncture points or myofascial trigger points

diode a tube that contains two electrodes that pass current in one direction

diplode a diathermy induction coil drum with flexible hinges

direct current (DC) electrical current that flows continually in one direction

disc herniation any disruption of the annular fibers of the intervertebral disc

disc prolapse an intervertebral disc herniation characterized by displacement of the nuclear material; the prolapse is contained by the outermost fibers of the disc

disc protrusion a distortion of the anatomic elements of the intervertebral disc without any internal disruption

discrimination the process of selectively targeting a specific form of nerve fiber

disease a definite morbid process that has a characteristic set of signs and symptoms

dislocation the displacement of a body part, especially bone

distraction the act of drawing or pulling along the long axis of a joint to the degree that the joint surfaces separate

dispersive electrode large electrode used to spread out electrical charge and decrease current density; often referred to as the ground electrode

distraction a state in which attention is diverted; a form of joint separation

direct current electrical current that always flows in the same direction (either positive or negative)

dorsal pertaining to the back or posterior aspect of a body part

dorsal horn the posterior portion of the gray matter of the spinal cord; the sensory portion of the spinal cord

dosage the product of intensity times duration

DuBois-Reymond law it is the variability of current density—not the absolute value of current density at any given moment—that acts as a stimulus to a muscle or a motor nerve

duration also referred to as pulse width; indicates the length of time from the beginning of one pulse of current to the end of the same pulse

duty cycle a method of measuring the interruption of current flow in pulsed ultrasound

dynorphin one of the naturally occurring opioid substances

dysfunction disturbance, impairment, or abnormality of the functioning of a body part or system

eccentric a type of muscle contraction that involves lengthening of the muscle; used to decelerate or absorb shock and control motion

ecchymosis an extravasation of blood under the skin

edema an accumulation of excessive fluid in the cells

efferent the conduction of a nerve impulse from the central nervous system to the periphery (motor)

effleurage a form of therapeutic massage that incorporates a light stroking without any attempt to move the deep muscles or tissues

electrical current the flow of electrons in an electrical circuit

electrical field a technique of heating tissues in shortwave diathermy in which the patient is part of the electrical circuit

electrical potential the difference in energy between charged particles at a higher and lower potential

electrical stimulation the application of electrical current to stimulate or depolarize nerve fibers, usually for therapeutic purposes

electricity a type of energy formed by the interaction of positive and negative charges

electroacupuncture analgesia the relief of pain by electrical stimulation of acupuncture points

electrode a surface from which an electrical current is discharged to a part of the body

electrodiagnosis the determination of functional states of various tissues and organs according to their responses to electrical current

electromagnetic or induction field a magnetic field that is not part of the circuit in which the patient is heated

electromagnetic spectrum the range of frequencies and wavelengths associated with radiant forms of energy

electromotive force (EMF) the result of a difference in electrical potential between two points that causes a flow of electricity, measured in volts

electromyography the detection and amplification of electrical signals generated by the muscle as it contracts

electron fundamental particles of matter possessing a negative electrical charge and extremely small mass

electrotherapy the application of electrical current for therapeutic purposes

electrostatic or condenser field an area between electrodes in which the patient is placed and becomes a part of a series circuit

emotional status the state of mental awareness, excitement

endogenous arising from or produced within the body

endogenous opiates naturally occurring opiates such as beta-endorphins

endorphin an opiatelike polypeptide produced in the brain and associated with natural pain relief

endurance tolerating or putting up with; to last or continue

enkephalin a group of pain-relieving neurotransmitters that inhibits the release of substance P

epiphysis the end of a long bone, originally separated from it by cartilage but later consolidated with it by ossification

episiotomy surgical excision of the vulvar orifice for obstetric purposes

erythema reddening of the skin caused by capillary dilation

erythema ab igne a redness of the skin caused by exposure to radiant heat

evaporation fluid loss by changing into vapor

evaluate to assess or quantify

evaluative pertaining to assessment

excitable capable of being excited; responding to a stimulus

exercise the performance of physical exertion for improvement of health or correction of dysfunction

exogenous originating externally; not produced within the body

exostosis bony growth that arises from the surface of a bone

extracapsular ligament a ligament found outside the joint capsule

extrusion a herniation of the intervertebral disc in which the nuclear material has burst through the posterior fibers and lies under the posterior ligament

exudate material that has escaped from blood vessels and been deposited in tissues; usually a result of inflammation

facet joints articular joints of the spine

facilitate to ease or assist

farad 1 farad is equal to the capacity of a condenser charged with 1 coulomb to give a difference of potential of 1 volt

faradic current an asymmetric alternating current

far ultraviolet ultraviolet radiation with a short wavelength, farthest from the visible spectrum

fatigue to tire or exhaust

fibrinogen a protein that is converted to fibrin

fibroblast a connective tissue cell responsible for the formation of the fibrous tissues of the body

fibrosis the formation of fibrous tissue during the injury or repair process

fibrous tissue the connective tissues of the body, tendons, ligaments, omenta, and so forth

first order pain the initial sensation of pain that is experienced; acute pain

flexion-distraction technique a method of treatment involving a specific treatment table; usually applied to intervertebral disc herniations

fluidotherapy a modality of dry heat that uses a finely dissolved solid suspended in a stream of moving air

fluoromethane a vapocoolant spray used to treat myofascial trigger points

fluorescence the capacity of substances to radiate when illuminated by a given wavelength; a light of a different wavelength than that of the irradiating source

fracture the breaking of a body part, especially a bone

free nerve endings pain-sensitive nerve endings

frequency the number of cycles or pulses per second; also called pulses per second (pps), cycles per second (cps), rate, pulse rate, and hertz (Hz)

frequency sweep a form of current modulation involving a variable or changing frequency

function the normal action of any body part

functional capacity assessment the evaluation of the action of body parts or systems

functional restoration the process of returning body parts or systems to a state of normal activity

galvanic current a nonpulsed, unidirectional (direct) current

gate theory of pain control a theory of pain control that states that stimulation of large, superficial sensory fibers will inhibit the perception of pain

general contraindication a situation or condition that renders the use of a certain procedure or treatment inadvisable under certain circumstances; treatment may, under some circumstances, continue with caution

generator an apparatus that converts mechanical energy into electrical energy

geriatric pertaining to the elderly

gravid pregnant

gravity reduction lumbar traction a form of traction that involves inversion and suspension of the patient

Grotthus-Draper law energy not absorbed by the tissues must be transmitted

ground a wire that makes an electrical connection with the earth

ground electrode large electrode used to spread out electrical charge and decrease current density; often referred to as the dispersive electrode

gym balls a large rubber ball that is used in the rehabilitation of balance and coordination; also referred to as Swiss balls

halo cast a cast applied to the shoulder containing metal bars that extend over the head and from which traction can be applied

Head's law pain produced by stimulation of viscera is felt in an area of the soma that corresponds to the organ affected

hematoma an area of swelling containing blood, usually clotted

hemodynamic events the series of events involving changes in capillary permeability and extravasation of fluid that accompanies the inflammatory process

herniation the protrusion of a body part through an opening; the protrusion of the nucleus pulposus through the annular portion of the intervertebral disc

hertz a unit for measuring frequency; equal to one pulse per second

Heuter-Volkmann theory an increase in pressure across a growing epiphyseal plate inhibits growth, whereas a decrease in pressure tends to accelerate growth

high voltage current current in which the waveform has an amplitude of greater than 150 volts with a relatively short pulse width

high voltage generator (HVG) an electrical stimulation device that uses a voltage in excess of 150 volts

high voltage pulsed stimulator (HVPS) an electrical stimulation device that uses a voltage in excess of 150 volts

histamine a powerful vasodilator

Hubbard tank an immersion tank for the whole body

hunting response a cyclic vasodilation that occurs in response to the application of cold; occurs within approximately 15 minutes

hydration to fill with fluid, especially water

hydrocollator a synthetic hot (170°F) or cold (0°F) gel used as an adjunctive modality to stimulate changes in tissue temperature

hydrocortisone an anti-inflammatory steroid sometimes used in phonophoresis or iontophoresis

hydrotherapy the application of both cryotherapy and thermotherapy techniques using water as the medium for heat transfer

hypalgesia a diminution or lessening of sensitivity to painful stimuli

hyper a state of excess, or more than normal

hyperalgesia an increased sensitivity to painful stimuli

hyperemia the presence of an increased amount of blood in a part of the body

hyperplasia an increase in the size of a tissue

hypermobile a state of excess movement

hyperstimulation a state of excess stimulation or excitement

hyperstimulation analgesia a method of pain control that uses a large amount of stimulus

hypo a state of less than normal

hypomobile a state of diminished movement

ice massage a method of therapy in which ice is rubbed on a body part

impedance the resistance of the tissue to the passage of electrical current, measured in ohms

immobilization to render incapable of being moved

impetigo a bacterial infection of the skin

indication the reason to prescribe a remedy or treatment procedure

indifferent or dispersive electrode large electrodes used to spread out electrical charge and decrease current density

induction the process by which a magnetizable body becomes magnetized when in a magnetic field, or by which an electromotive force is created in a circuit by varying the magnetic field linked with the circuit

induction electrodes electrical current is passed through a coil that in turn gives off eddy currents of electromagnetic energy; this energy is absorbed by the tissues and heat is produced by tissue resistance

inflammation the condition that tissues enter into as a result of injury

informed consent the ability of a patient to make choices based on an understanding of the relevant consequences of that choice on oneself and others

infrared that portion of the electromagnetic spectrum that is associated with thermal changes

infrared modalities those therapeutic devices that use some form of infrared energy

instability not stable; incapable of resisting normal physiologic stresses

insulation the protection of the body or a body part with a nonconducting electrical medium to prevent the transfer of energy

intensity refers to the amount of energy applied in a given treatment such as ultrasound or electrical stimulation

interferential current (IFC) an electrical stimulator that employs two biphasic sinusoidal waves that are slightly out of phase with each other (medium frequency currents)

intermittent traction a form of traction involving forces that are alternately applied and released

intermolecular vibration a movement between molecules that creates friction and results in the formation of heat within the tissues

interneurons neurons contained entirely in the central nervous system; they serve as relay stations

interrupted current an electrical current that is not delivered in a continuous manner; a surged current

interpulse interval the interval from the end of one pulse of current to the beginning of the next pulse, measured in microseconds

interrupted current a flow of electricity that is frequently and regularly turned on and off

intersegmental traction a form of traction involving mechanical rollers that move up and down along the paraspinal structures

inverse square law the intensity of radiation at any distance from the radiating source is directly proportional to the inverse of the square of the distance between the source of energy and the target

iodine a chemical that is often used with iontophoresis in the treatment of scars and adhesions

ion an electrically charged particle

ionization the process by which neutral atoms or molecules become positively or negatively charged

iontophoresis the use of constant direct current (galvanic) to drive ions into and through the skin

irradiation exposure to some form of radiation

ischemia local anemia due to some type of functional or mechanical obstruction to circulation

isokinetic a form of exercise or muscle contraction that involves a constant or steady speed

isometric a form of muscle contraction that involves no change in muscle length

isotonic a form of exercise or muscle contraction that involves a constant or steady force

joint capsule the ligamentous structure that surrounds the synovial joint

joint contracture a pathologic state involving immobilization of a joint by muscle spasm

joint play that portion of joint movement that is not under active control (*e.g.,* long-axis extension of the interphalangeal joints)

joule a unit of electrical energy equivalent to the work expended when 1 ampere flows for 1 second against a resistance of 1 ohm

Joule's law heat is produced in direct proportion to the square of the current strength; heat produced by a given amount of current is directly proportional to the resistance of the conductor; and the heat produced is directly proportional to the duration of current flow

Karya gum a material that is used to coat self-adhesive electrodes

keloids hypertrophy of a scar

keratin a fibrous protein that forms the chemical basis of the epidermis

keratosis a horny growth such as a wart or callous

kilovolt a unit of electrical potential or electromotive force that represents 1000 volts

Kirchoff's law the greatest level of heat is produced in the area of greatest current density

kneading a type of therapeutic massage that incorporates pressing, grasping, and wringing of a part of a muscle or muscle group

Kromayer lamp a trade name for a hot quartz ultraviolet lamp

lamina a thin, flat plate or layer

latent period that period of time between the initiation of a stimulus and the body's response

lead-zirconium-titanate (PZT) a man-made crystal that is used in ultrasound devices

Lennox-Hill brace an orthopedic appliance used to stabilize the knee

leukocytes white blood cells

lidocaine a chemical used for analgesia, often used with iontophoresis

ligament a fibrous connective tissue structure that connects one bone to another

locomotor system the system that provides motion to the body; the neuromusculoskeletal system

longitudinal wave that portion of the ultrasound wave that travels from the ultrasound head to the patient

LoTENS treatment technique that involves electrical stimulation of acupuncture points to achieve pain relief; also referred to as acupuncturelike TENS

low voltage current current in which the waveform has a maximal amplitude of less than 150 volts

luminous the property to give off light; those infrared lamps that give off light or glow

lysozyme an enzyme that is capable of breaking apart structures and chemicals

macrophage a large mononuclear cell that is responsible for destroying and ingesting bacteria and cellular debris

magnetic field a technique of heating the tissues seen in shortwave diathermy in which the patient is not part of the electrical circuit

magnetron a diode vacuum tube used to generate power in microwave diathermy units

malignancy the state of being malignant or cancerous

malingering the willful and deliberate feigning of symptoms or exaggeration of symptoms of illness or injury for a conscious gain

manipulation a form of manual treatment directed at the synovial joints involving a quick thrust that is beyond the patient's ability to resist; specifically used to restore normal joint mobility

manual traction a form of traction that involves the application of manual forces

margination a part of the inflammatory process that involves capillary dilation, slowing of the blood stream, and an accumulation of leukocytes along the margins of the vessels

massage the act of rubbing, kneading, or stroking the superficial parts of the body with the hand to restore movement and circulation or to break up adhesions

McGill Pain Questionnaire a pain measurement instrument used to quantify and qualify pain

microwave diathermy a form of deep heating that uses a portion of the radio wave spectrum; sometimes used for tumor eradication

mechanical effects one of the effects of ultrasonic treatment resulting from the vibration of molecules

mechanoreceptor a sensory nerve that is activated by some form of mechanical stimulus such as pressure, movement, or distortion

mechanotherapy the application of some type of mechanical therapy

mecholyl an ointment with 0.025% methacholine and 10% salicylate; an effective vasodilator that is used with phonophoresis for a variety of vascular conditions and neurovascular deficits

mediator to effect something by means of an intermediary substance

megahertz (MHz) a frequency of 1 million cycles per second

melanin a group of dark brown or black pigments that occur in the superficial tissues

meniscus a cartilaginous structure found on the synovial fringes of some joints (*e.g.*, the knee)

meridian the pathway of energy flow that is used in acupuncture

metabolites waste products of metabolism

metal implant any metal device placed within the tissues

metatarsal referring to one of the bones of the foot

minimal erythemal dose (MED) the amount of time of exposure to ultraviolet light necessary to cause a faint erythema 24 hours after exposure

microamp one millionth of an ampere; the unit of electrical current used in microcurrent stimulators

microamperage stimulation devices that form of electrical stimulator that uses a subthreshold current, measured in microamperes; usually associated with pain control and tissue healing

microcoulomb that quantity of electricity transferred by a current of one thousandth of an ampere in 1 second

microcurrent stimulator an electrical stimulator that is used to stimulate healing and pain relief; uses a current with subthreshold intensity measured in microamps

microsecond one millionth of a second; used in measuring the pulse width of most electrical stimulators

mild injury may or may not require treatment; the person is able to continue with most, if not all, activities of daily living; treatment is brief and usually successful

mild pain does cause some suffering and rarely interferes with the person's emotional status; any changes are usually temporary

milliampere one thousandth of an ampere; used in measuring the current intensity of most electrical stimulators

milliamps per second (MAS) a radiologic unit derived by multiplying the number of electrons applied to the cathode of an x-ray tube by the exposure time in seconds

millisecond one thousandth of a second

minimal erythemal dose (MED) the least amount of ultraviolet radiation necessary to produce erythema

minimal injury an injury that usually does not require treatment; the person is able to continue with all activities of daily living and the condition resolves quickly

minimal pain does not cause suffering and does not interfere with the person's emotional status; the injured individual usually does not seek professional help

mobilization the methods involved in improving motion in a joint

modality a method of therapy or use of a therapeutic agent

mode the method or manner in which something is done

moderate injury typically requires treatment; some activities of daily living are affected; treatment usually takes weeks to a few months

moderate pain causes suffering and may interfere with emotional status; usually prompts a person to seek treatment

modify to change or alter

modulation refers to any alteration in the magnitude or any variation in the duration of an electrical current

moist heat a superficial thermal agent; usually applied with dampened cloth bags containing silica

monocyte a large mononuclear leukocyte

monophasic having a single phase or cycle

monophasic current a current in which the direction of flow remains the same; also known as direct current

monopolar having a single polarity or charge; refers to direct current devices

morphine a product of opium that produces analgesia

morphology the study of the configuration or structure of the body

motor level stimulus (MLS) a level of electrical intensity that is associated with depolarization of motor nerves and subsequent muscle contraction

motor point the point where a motor nerve enters a muscle; identified by a reduction in electrical skin resistance

motion unit the functional unit of the spine consisting of two adjacent vertebral segments

motor neuron a nerve cell body in the central nervous system that is responsible for muscle contraction

motor unit a motor neuron and the muscle fibers that it innervates

muscle energy procedure a type of manual treatment procedure that employs the patient's active muscle contraction as part of the therapy

musculoskeletal referring to the muscles and the skeleton

myelin a fatty material that surrounds the axons of certain nerve fibers

myelinated fibers those nerve fibers that are protected by a myelin sheath

myofascial refers to the fascia surrounding and separating muscle tissue

myofascial pain a type of referred pain associated with trigger points

myofascial trigger points a focus of hyperirritability in a muscle which, when provoked, can refer pain, paraesthesia, and/or autonomic symptoms to an area that is specific for the muscle

myofascitis inflammation of the myofascial tissue

myositis ossificans inflammation of muscle tissue with resulting bony formation within the muscle

naloxone a narcotic antagonist

necrosis the pathologic death of one of more cells, or of a tissue or organ

nerve root impingement abnormal encroachment of some tissue into the space occupied by the nerve root

nerve terminals the end of a nerve fiber

neuroma a growth or tumor arising from the nervous system

neuromodulation the process of changing or altering the nervous system

neuromusculoskeletal system referring to the nerves, muscles, and skeleton

neuropathy a disorder affecting a portion of the nervous system

neurotransmitter a chemical substance that allows the passage of information between adjacent neurons; some neurotransmitters enhance nerve activity (excitatory) whereas others delay nerve activity (inhibitory)

neutrophil a mature white blood cell

nociceptor a neuron that is stimulated by injury; a receptor for pain

nonluminous referring to an infrared lamp that does not glow or emit light

nonsteroidal anti-inflammatory medications (NSAIDs) a type of pharmaceutical used to reduce inflammation

norepinephrine a neurotransmitter that may enhance pain

noxious painful, unpleasant

noxious-level stimulus (NLS) a level of electrical intensity that is associated with depolarization of nociceptors; a painful electrical stimulus used to reduce pain

nucleus pulposus the central portion of the intervertebral disc

nutrient essential or nonessential food substances

nutritional status refers to the nutritional condition of a patient

objective pertaining to something that can be easily seen by others

occupational therapy a form of treatment directed at restoring an injured individual's ability to perform work

ohm a measurement of resistance to electrical current

Ohm's law the current in an electrical circuit is directly proportional to the voltage and inversely proportional to the resistance (*i.e.*, I = v / r)

open circuit an electrical circuit that is not complete or not closed

onset the beginning or start

oscillating current an alternating current with either a constant wave amplitude or a gradually diminishing amplitude

oscilloscope a device used to depict the nature and form of electrical waves

oscillator a device that produces electrical oscillations or waves of a particular frequency

osteomalacia a softening of the bones associated with progressive deformity

osteoporosis a condition associated with demineralization of the bones

outcome measures tools that are used to evaluate or assess the effectiveness of treatment

output the quantity emitted or produced during a specific period of time

overuse syndrome injury to a tissue by subjecting it to an activity that it is not able to withstand, either it is too vigorous or is extended over a period of time

pad electrodes capacitor type electrodes used with shortwave diathermy

pain a specific response to tissue damage or the perception of tissue damage

pain drawing a pain measurement tool; a picture of a person used to illustrate the location of a patient's pain

pain-spasm-pain cycle a physiologic cycle involving muscle spasm and resultant pain

palliative having the ability to reduce the severity of symptoms

paraffin bath a combination of paraffin and mineral oil (melting temperature 126°F) that is used to increase the temperature of superficial tissue; commonly used in the hands and feet

parameter an arbitrary constant, factor, or measurement

paraesthesia abnormal sensation; a sensation of itching, tingling, or pins and needles

paroxysmal cold hemoglobinuria a vascular condition associated with an abnormal reaction to cold exposure

passive being acted upon by external agents; characterized by lack of activity

passive range of motion that portion of the joint movement that can be initiated by someone other than the patient

pathology that branch of medicine that concerns itself with the study of disease; the disease process

pattern theory a theory of pain perception that states pain may be perceived when the stimulus conforms to a particular pattern

peak current the greatest intensity of a pulse of electrical current

penetration the ability to pierce or enter

percussion a type of massage therapy that uses a tapping or thumping stroke; tapotement

percutaneous any method that incorporates piercing the skin, as in percutaneous electrical nerve stimulation

periarticular the tissue surrounding a synovial joint

period the time required for one cycle of alternating current to pass through all of its positive and negative cycles

peripheral distant from the center; pertaining to the outer or external portion

petrissage a massage technique that uses a deep, kneading stroke; consists of repeatedly grasping and releasing the tissues with the hands

periosteum the connective tissue covering of the bones

Pfluger's law a nerve tract is stimulated when catelectrotonus develops (negative pole) but not when anelectrotonus develops (positive pole)

phase duration the time of a particular pulse of current; the pulse width

phonophoresis the process of driving some type of medication into the subcutaneous tissues by ultrasound

phoresis refers to the migration of ions through a membrane

phosphorescence the induced luminescence that persists after the irradiation causing it has ceased

photokeratitis an inflammation of the eyes caused by exposure to ultraviolet light

photometer an instrument used to measure light intensity

physiatry the study of physiotherapeutics; the treatment of disease by physical means

physical therapy the application of specific modalities such as heat, light, water, ultrasound, and electricity for the treatment of disease; a specific form of health sciences

piezoelectric effect the vibration of a crystal that results from passing an electrical current through it; the transformation of mechanical energy into electrical energy

pituitary gland one of the endocrine glands found at the base of the brain

plexus a network or interlacement; usually refers to a collection of nerves or blood vessels

plica a thickened portion of synovium; a synovial fold

polarity the orientation of electrons or charged particles based on their positive or negative charge

polarize to arrange in a specific order; to separate in different directions

polymodal nociceptors small unmyelinated sensory fibers that respond to a variety of stimuli such as deep pressure and temperature (C fibers)

polyphasic current current that contains three or more grouped phases in a single phase; used in interferential and "Russian" stimulation

positional traction a form of mechanical traction using certain body positions

potential in electrotherapy, refers to the difference in electrical energy from one point to another; measured in volts

pps pulses per second; synonymous with hertz

primary main; first in a series of sequence

prime mover a muscle or muscle group that is primarily responsible for a given movement; an agonist

prognosis a prediction or conclusion regarding the course or outcome of a disease or treatment process

pronation the act of turning the palm downward; a downward positioning of a limb

prone a face-down position

propagation to multiply or reproduce

proprioception the sensation of body awareness

proprioceptive neuromuscular facilitation (PNF) a manual therapeutic procedure that is designed to re-establish coordination

proprioceptor a sensory nerve that provides information regarding joint movement, pressure, and muscle tone

prostaglandin substances that are found during tissue injury; they act as powerful vasodilators and produce erythema; aspirin is thought to inhibit their production

proteolytic an enzyme that is capable of breaking down protein

protocol the rules or guidelines of a treatment regimen

provocative serving to stimulate or aggravate

psychological refers to the mind or to mental state

psychological overlay mental or emotional factors that may complicate a clinical picture

psychosocial refers to mental, emotional, and personal factors

pulsatile current an electric current that is delivered in pulses

pulse charge the total accumulation of electrical current in a tissue

pulse duration the length of time from the beginning of one phase of an electrical pulse to the end of the same phase; usually measured in microseconds

pulsed current a type of electrical current that is delivered in pieces or pulses

pulsed duty cycle a modification of ultrasonic energy used to reduce any accumulation of heat

pulsed ultrasound a method of administering ultrasound in which the production of sound waves is intermittent

pulse width refers to the pulse duration

Q-tip electrode a type of electrode that uses a moistened Q-tip or cotton swab; usually found with the microcurrent stimulation devices

quadripolar an electrode placement technique; refers to the use of two bipolar currents found with interferential current stimulators

quality the characteristics of a thing that determines its value, place, or worth

radiation the process of emitting energy from some source in the form of waves; a method of heat transfer

radicular radiating or spreading

radiculitis inflammation of a nerve root

ramping a modulation used with a surged or interrupted current in which the current builds gradually to some maximal amplitude; used for patient comfort

range of motion the degree or arc of movement of a particular joint or tissue

raphe nucleus a part of the brain known to inhibit the transmission of pain impulses

rate of rise how quickly a waveform reaches its maximal amplitude

Raynaud's disease a pathologic condition of the blood vessels of the hand that is associated with exposure to cold

reaction of degeneration the change in muscle response to electrical current; seen in nerve injuries

reactivation to make active or functional again

reciprocal a complimentary action of two opposing entities

reciprocal inhibition a physiologic principle stating that activation of one muscle or muscle group will produce inhibition of the reciprocal (antagonist) muscle or muscle group

reciprocal mode a setting on an electrical stimulator that allows an alternating stimulus to reciprocal or antagonist muscle groups

recruitment to enlist or add to; the activation of additional nerve or muscle fibers

rectified corrected; purified; changing an alternating current to a direct current

referred pain pain that is felt at a distance from the lesion

reflection the bending back of energy (light or sound waves) from a surface that it strikes

refraction the change in direction that occurs when energy passes from one medium to another

refractory period the period of depolarization of a nerve prior to its return to a normal resting state

rehabilitation the process of restoring to a former state

relative referring to, relating to, or qualifying

relative contraindication a condition that serves as a precaution for treatment

remodeling to make over or new again

remodeling stage that time period following an injury during which the body attempts to restore tissues to their former condition

repolarization restoring the polarity of a nerve or muscle fiber

resistance opposition to the flow of electrical current, measured in ohms

resistor a device or substance that inhibits the flow of electrical current

resonance an inherent state of vibratory activity

rheobase the minimal amount of electrical current necessary to cause stimulation

rheostat a device for regulating a current by means of varying electrical resistance

rheumatoid arthritis a pathologic condition associated with inflammation of joints

RICE rest, ice, compression, and elevation; the classic or standard treatment for the acute stage of injury

rocker board a therapeutic device that is used to establish balance and coordination

Russian stimulation a form of electrical stimulation associated with increasing muscle strength

SAID specific adaptation to imposed demand; a principal concept in rehabilitation

salicylate a salt or ester of salicylic acid

scar a mark left on the skin after a wound or injury has healed

scleroderma a pathologic hardening of the skin

sclerotogenous pain pain originating from sclerotogenous structures

sclerotome a segment of bone innervated by a spinal segment

second order pain pain that is sensed or perceived after the acute phase; not first or primary

sedate to quiet or put to sleep

sensitization the process of rendering a cell receptive to stimuli

sensory referring to that portion of the nervous system responsible for incoming impulses

sepsis a state of disease involving the presence of toxic substances such as bacteria in the blood stream

sequestration a herniation of the intervertebral disc in which nuclear material may extrude through the posterior fibers of the annulus and through the posterior ligament; free floating fragment of intervertebral disc in the spinal canal

serotonin a neurotransmitter found in the vesicles in nerve endings; in low levels, serotonin may assist in analgesia; in higher concentrations, it may produce pain

severe injury this is a life-threatening, potentially mutilating, disfiguring, or otherwise horrible injury

severe pain a horrible pain that causes intense suffering and, by itself, functionally disables the patient

severity refers to the degree or intensity of pain or injury

SHARP swelling, heat, altered function, redness and pain; the acronym used to describe the symptoms associated with the acute stage

shortwave diathermy a form of deep heating therapy using a particular type of electromagnetic energy

sine wave (sinusoidal) a particular type of waveform

sinusoidal current an electrical current using a sinusoidal waveform

sleeve test a procedure used to determine the amount of ultraviolet radiation to be used

soft tissue refers to the muscles, fascia, and connective tissues

somatic refers to the musculoskeletal system

somatosensory refers to sensations involving the musculoskeletal system

sonation the process of treating with ultrasonic energy

space plate an air-spaced condenser-field applicator used in shortwave diathermy

spasm an involuntary, sustained muscular contraction

spatial refers to distance or space

specificity theory a theory of pain perception that states pain may only be perceived by specific nerve fibers

spectrum the charted band of wavelengths of electromagnetic energy

splint an appliance used to fix or stabilize an injured body part

spondylolisthesis a forward displacement of one vertebra over another

spondylosis degeneration of a vertebra

spondylotherapy the application of manual procedures to the spine

sprain an injury to a ligament

spray and stretch a therapeutic procedure directed at myofascial trigger points

square wave a pulse of electrical current that uses a square or rectangular waveform

stamina the ability to resist fatigue or tiring

stabilize to make firm or stable

stellate ganglion a ganglion formed by the first thoracic ganglion and the inferior cervical ganglion

stenosis a hardening or narrowing of a vessel or canal

stimulus produced analgesia (SPA) pain relief that is produced by stimulation of the nervous system

strain an injury to a muscle

strength-duration curve an illustration of the relationship between current intensity and current duration in causing depolarization of nerve fibers

subacute the stage of injury that follows the acute or early period; associated with fragile, easily reinjured tissue

subdermal below the skin or dermis

subjective pertaining to or perceived only by the affected individual

subluxation a state of less than normal position or function of adjacent bony segments

substance P a pain producing neurotransmitter thought to activate the small diameter nociceptors

substantia gelatinosa an area in the dorsal horn of the spinal cord associated with the "gate theory of pain control"

subthreshold a stimulus that is inadequate to elicit a response

summation the result of an addition of stimuli or effects

summation of contractions shortening of muscle myofilaments caused by increasing the frequency of muscle membrane depolarization

summation principle sequential stimuli that may be individually inadequate to evoke a response collectively are able to induce a nerve stimulus

superficial referring to the upper or outer portion of the body; near the surface

superimposition the process of placing one thing directly over another; used in interferential current

supination the act of turning the palm upward; an upward positioning of a limb

supine a recumbent face-up patient position

suppress to put an end to; to stop

surge an interrupted electrical current that gradually rises and falls

sustained traction a type of mechanical traction that uses a continuous or constant force

switch rate a control setting on an electrical stimulator that permits the alternate activation of two different sets of electrodes

symptom any evidence of a patient's disease or condition

synapse the junction point between two neurons, across which a nerve impulse passes

synaptic transmission the process by which a nerve impulse crosses the junction between two neurons

synovial joint a joint between two bones that is lined with synovial fluid

synovium the lining of a synovial joint

tapotement a therapeutic massage technique using a series of brisk strokes or blows in rapid succession; also called percussion

T cell an internuncial (relay) neuron found in lamina V of the spinal cord

temporal refers to time

tenderness a symptom characterized by sensitivity to pressure or contact

TENS transcutaneous electrical nerve stimulation

tetany a smooth, sustained muscle contraction

therapy the treatment of an illness or disease

thermal pertains to heat

thermal energy energy that produces or extracts heat

thermopane an insulating layer of water next to the skin

thermotherapy the therapeutic application of heat to treat pathology or disease

threshold the point where a stimulus begins to produce a response; the minimal stimulus necessary to elicit a response

thrombophlebitis inflammation of a vein with a blood clot formed within a blood vessel

tolerable the ability to withstand or put up with

total current the amount of current that is delivered during treatment

traction the process of applying tension to a body segment to separate the parts

transcerebral the application of electrical current across the cranium

transcutaneous across the skin

transcutaneous electrical nerve stimulation (TENS) the process of delivering an electrical current through the skin via surface electrodes

transducer a device that changes energy from one type to another (*e.g.,* an ultrasound head)

transformer a device used to change the voltage in electrical currents

transmission the process of transferring or exchanging

transudate the fluid that escapes from pores or tissues following an injury

transverse wave one of the waves emitted by an ultrasound unit

twitch muscle contraction a single muscle contraction caused by one isolated depolarization

trigger point a local area of hyperirritability in a muscle that when provoked, refers pain, paraesthesia, and/or autonomic symptoms to an area that is specific for the muscle

twin-peaked wave an electrical pulse that uses a wave with two peaks; usually associated with high voltage currents

ultrasound a portion of the acoustic spectrum that is located above the audible sound

ultraviolet that portion of the electromagnetic spectrum associated with chemical changes; it is located adjacent to the violet portion of the visible light spectrum

uncomplicated injury a confined or singular injury or injury complex that closely matches the mechanism of injury

unstable not secure or firm

vacuum electrode a type of electrode with which suction is used to secure it to the patient; associated with interferential current stimulators

vasoconstriction a narrowing of the blood vessels

vapocoolant a fine mist cooling agent administered to distract prior to stretching a muscle; may also be used to temporarily reduce pain

vasodilation a widening or opening of the blood vessels

vectoring the change in direction of electrical current used in interferential current

velocity the state of moving quickly; the speed of movement

vibration a shaking massage technique that incorporates a fine tremulous movement

viscera refers to the internal body organs

viscoelastic a property of connective tissue that provides both viscous and elastic responses

Visual Analog Scale (VAS) a pain measurement tool that asks the patient to grade the severity of pain between zero and 10

vocational therapy a type of treatment directed at retraining an injured individual for a different type of work

volt the electromotive force that produces movement of electrons

watt a measure of electrical power; watts = volts × amperes

wave one wavelength; a single electrical impulse

waveform the shape of an electrical current as displayed on an oscilloscope

wavelength the distance from one point in a propagating wave to the same point in the next wave

Wedensky inhibition a phenomenon in which the continuous stimulation of a nerve by a medium frequency electrical current leads to inhibition of painful impulses; thought to be due to fatigue of the sensory nerve or some form of nerve block

wobble board a therapeutic device that is used to establish balance and coordination

Wolff's law a physiologic law that states that the internal architecture of a bone is determined by the external pressures exerted on it

Wood's filter a screen that permits ultraviolet light to be transmitted; used in detecting ring worm

work hardening a rehabilitation technique designed to re-establish an injured individual's ability to work

zinc a chemical used with iontophoresis and phonophoresis

Figure credits
. . . .

Figure 2.8
From Melzack R. The McGill pain questionnaire: Major properties and scoring methods. Pain 1975; 1:275.

Figures 3.2 and 3.3
From Travell JG, Simons DG. Myofascial pain and dysfunction: The trigger point manual: The upper extremities (vol 1) and The lower extremities (vol 2). Baltimore: Williams & Wilkins, 1983 (vol 1) 1992 (vol 2).

Figure 4.1
Adapted from Prentice WE. Therapeutic modalities in sports medicine. St Louis: Times Mirror Mosby, 1986.

Figures 4.8 and 4.9
From Travell JG, Simmons DG. Myofascial pain and dysfunction: The trigger point manual: The upper extremities (vol 1) and The lower extremities (vol 2). Baltimore: Williams & Wilkins, 1983 (vol 1) 1992 (vol 2).

Figures 4.10, 7.2, 7.3, 7.10, 9.6 and 9.8
Couresy of Chattanooga Group, Inc., Hixson, Tennessee

Figure 9.1
Adapted from Natchev E. A manual on autotraction treatment for low back pain. Sundsvall, Tryckcribolaget, 1984. In Hooper PD. Preventing low back pain. Baltimore: Williams & Wilkins, 1992.

Figures 10.1 to 10.15
Courtesy of Anabolic Laboratories, Irvine, California

Appendix A
McGill Pain Questionnaire
From Melzack R. The McGill pain questionnaire: Major properties and scoring mehtods. Pain 1975;1:275.

Oswestry Low Back Pain Disability Questionnaire
From Fairbanks J, Davies J. The Oswestry low back pain disability questionnaire. Physiotherapy 1980;66:271.

Roland Morris Pain Questionnaire
From Roland M, Morris R. Study of natural history of back pain. Part I: Development of reliable and sensitive measure of disability in low back pain. Spine 1983;8:141.

Becker's Red Flags
Adapted from Becker GE. Chronic pain, depression, and the injured worker. PsychiatryAnn 1991;21:1.

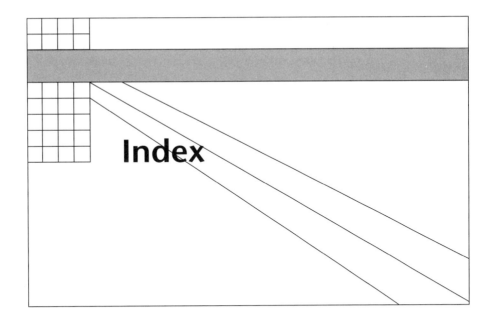

Index

Page numbers in *italics* denote figures.